MW00929867

Sometimes
the
Smallest
Things take up
the most room
in your
Heart.

Winnie the Pooh

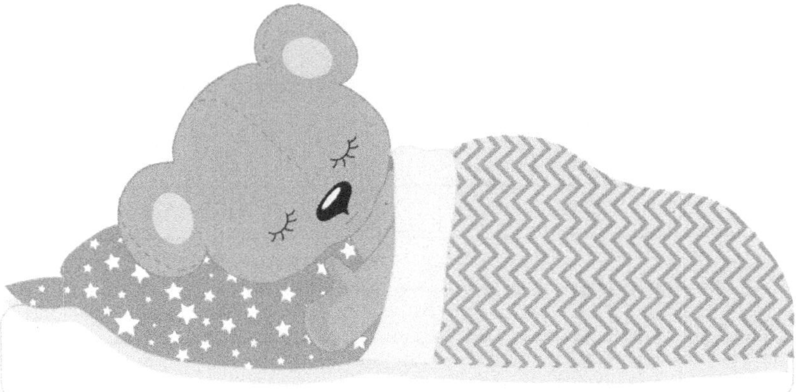

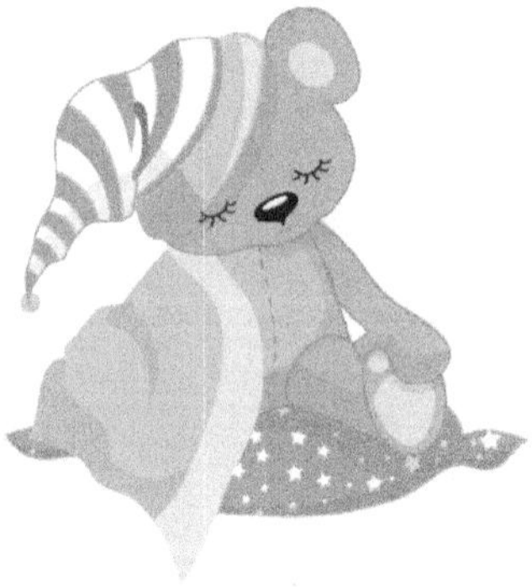

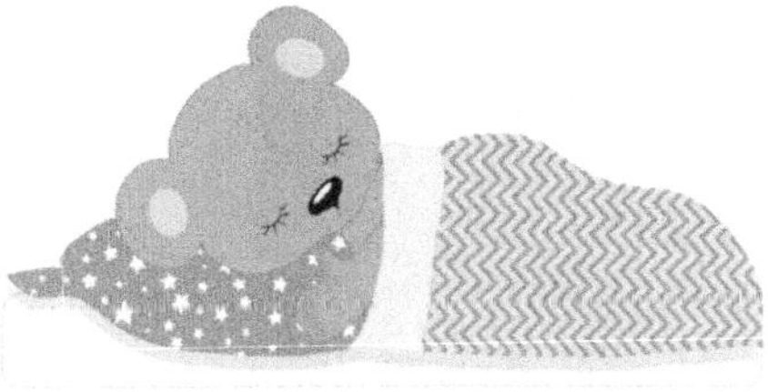

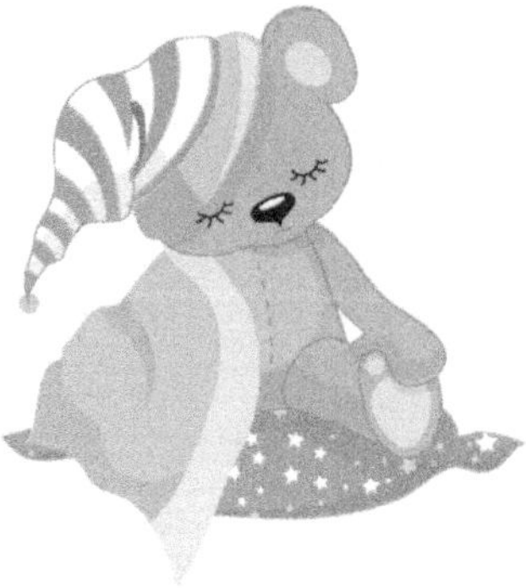

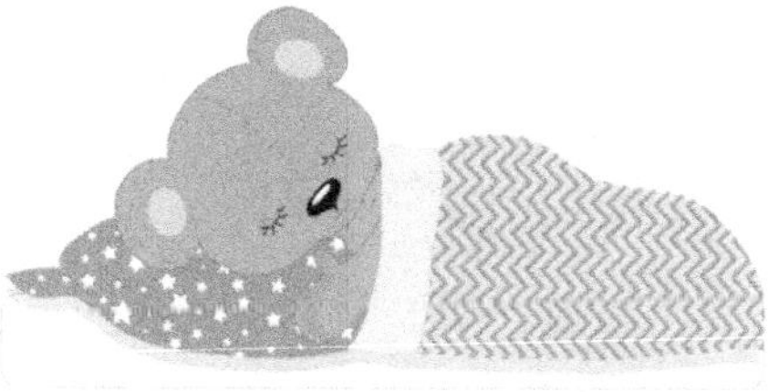

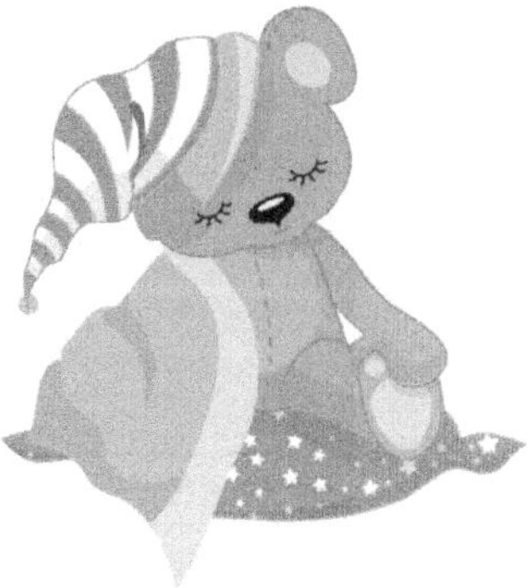

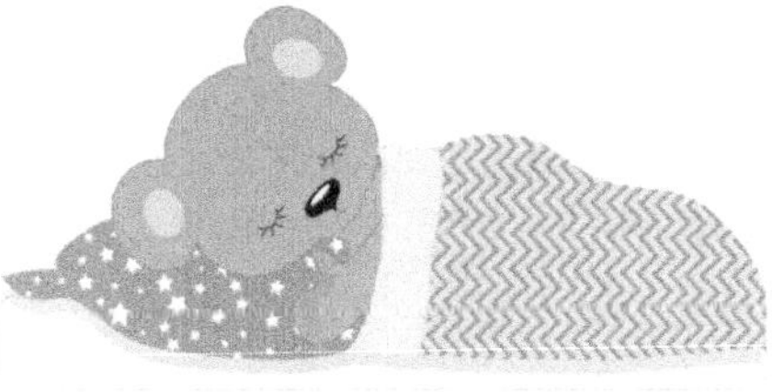

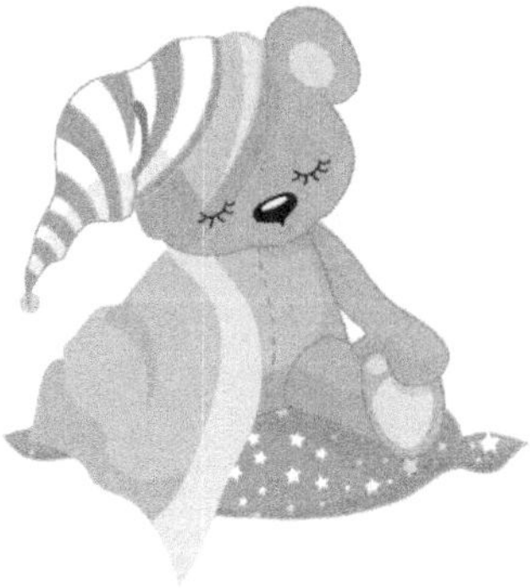

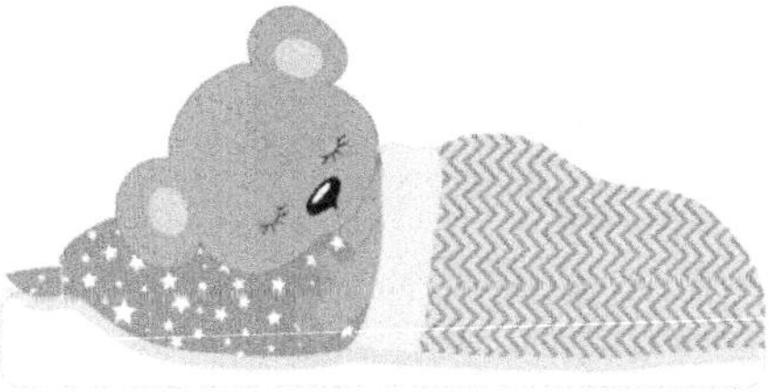

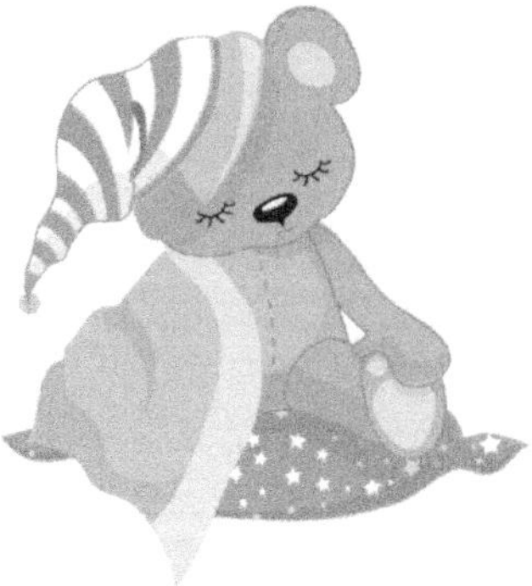

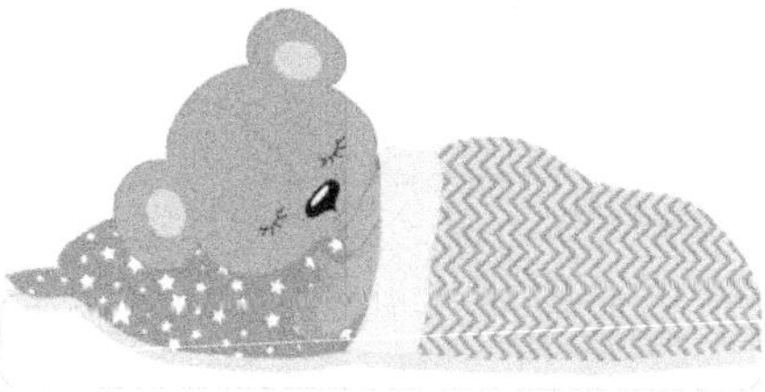

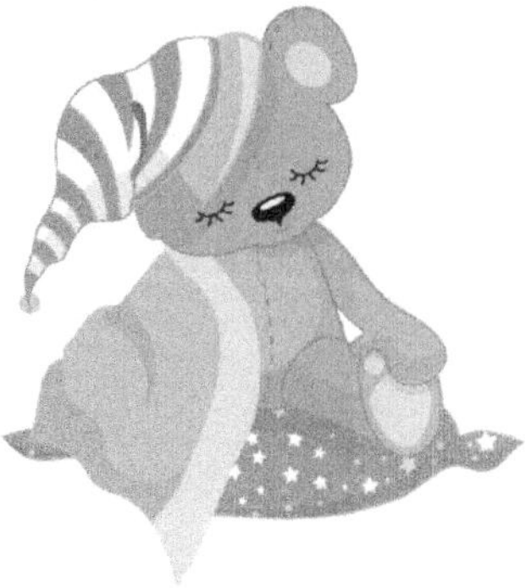

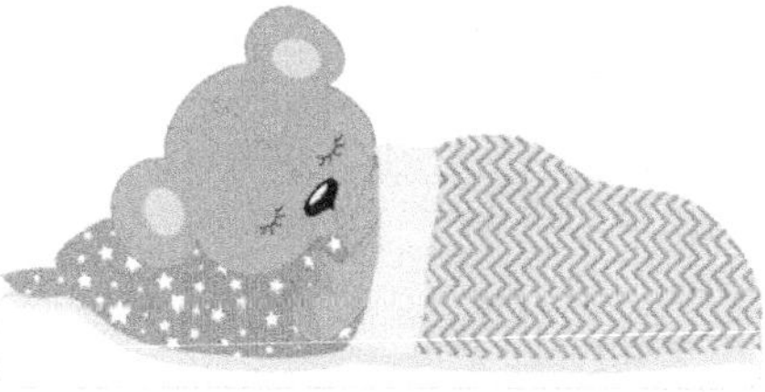

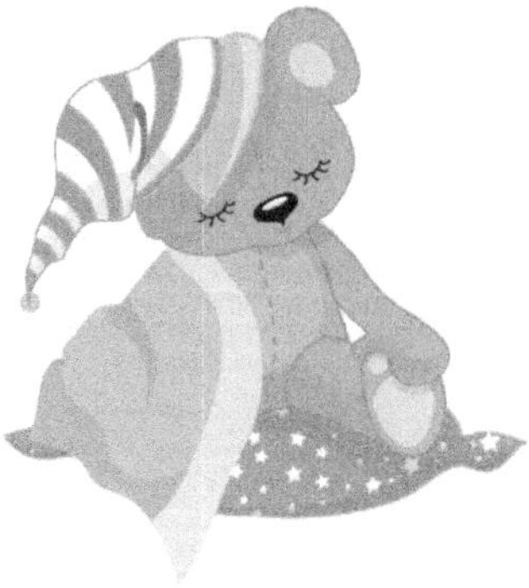

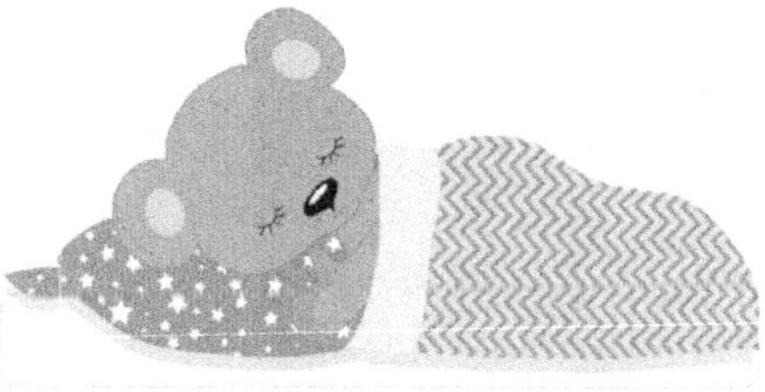

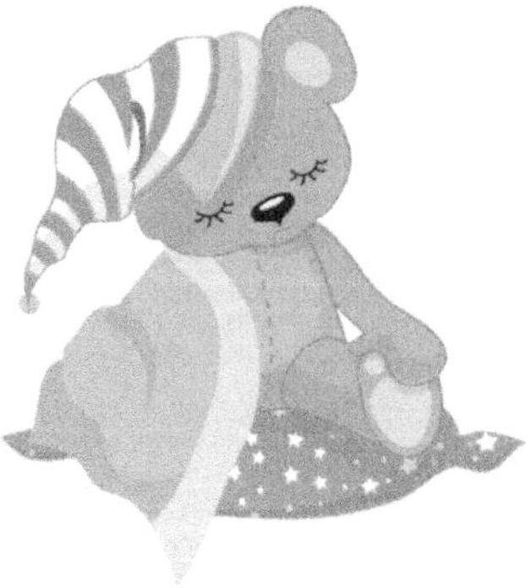

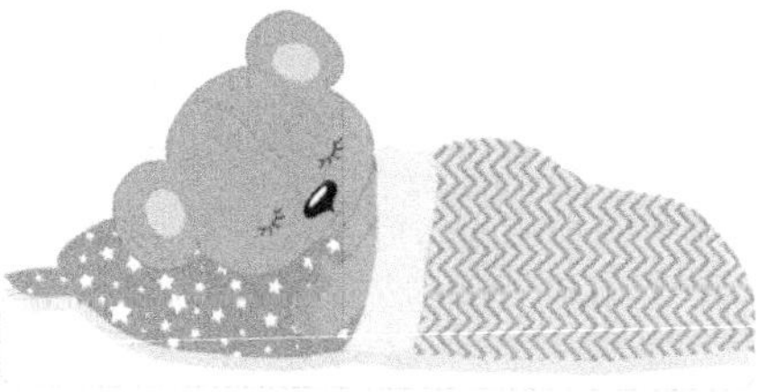

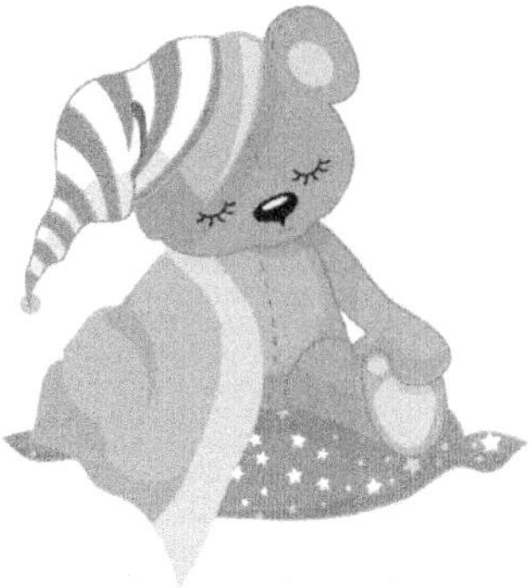

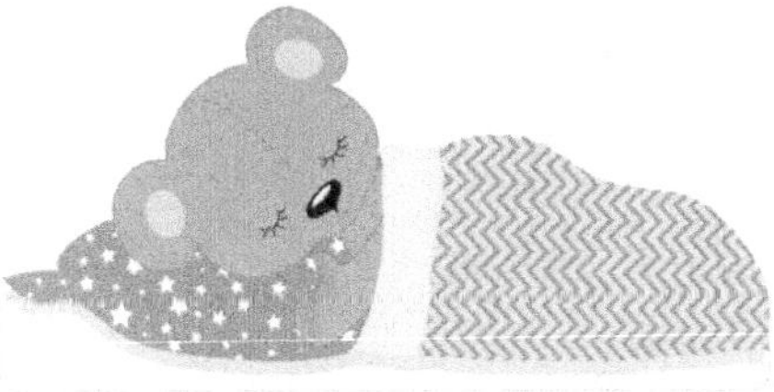

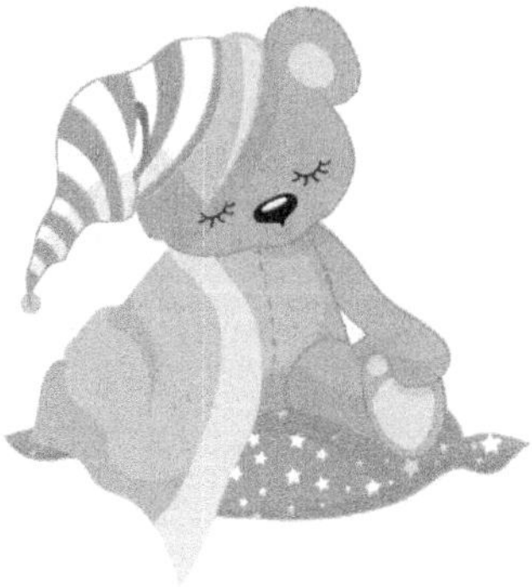

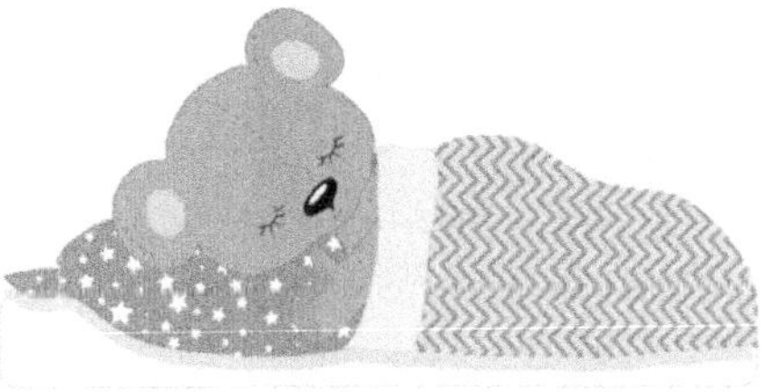

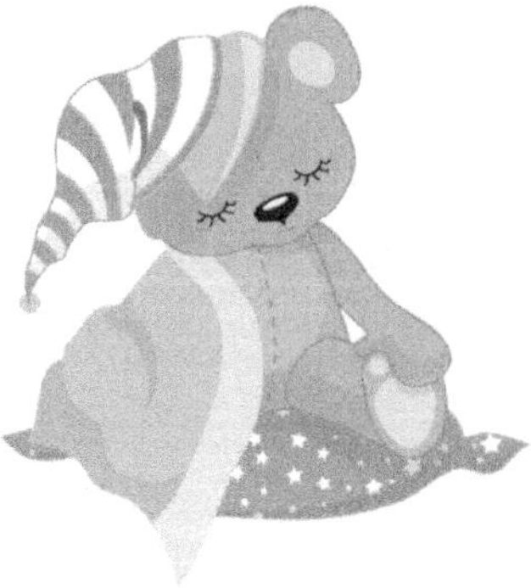

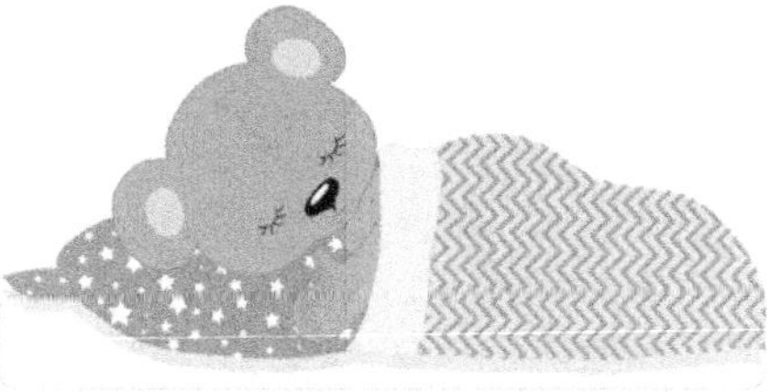

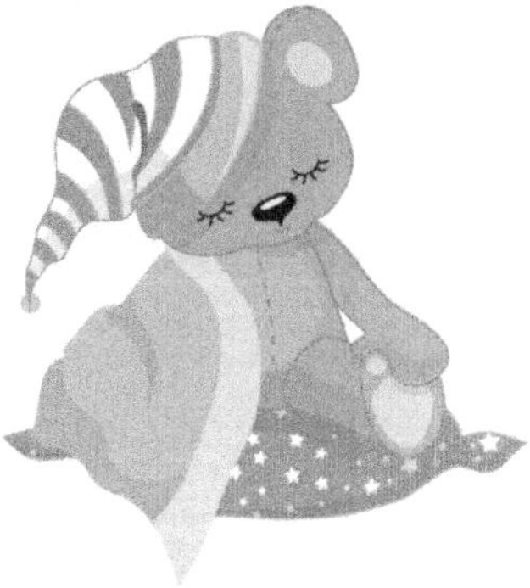

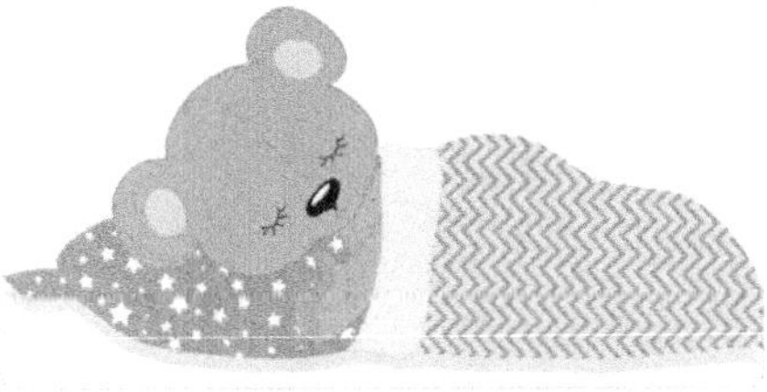

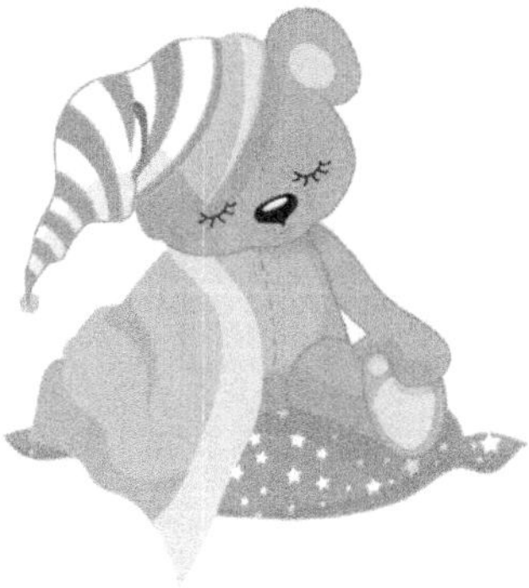

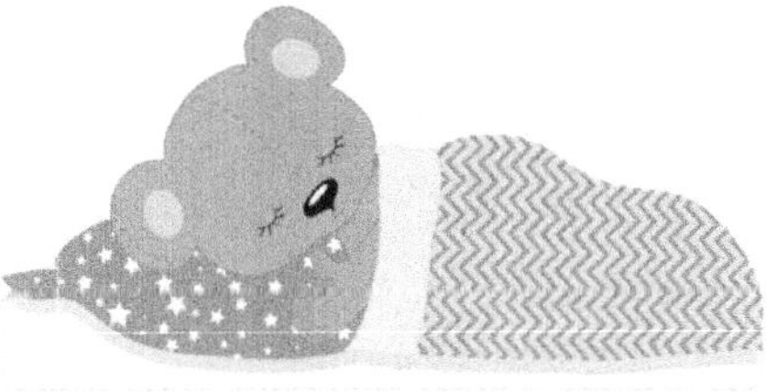

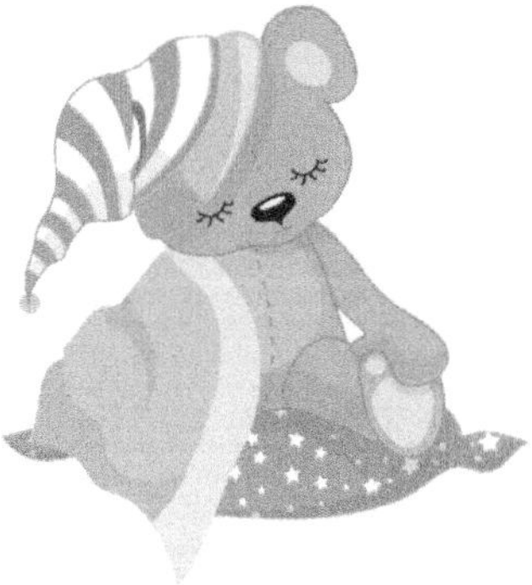

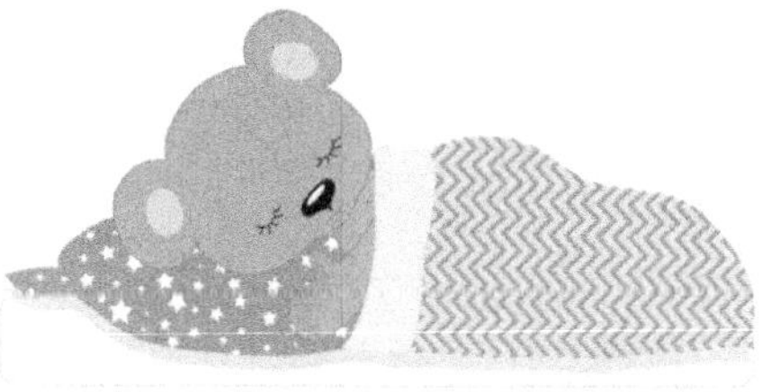

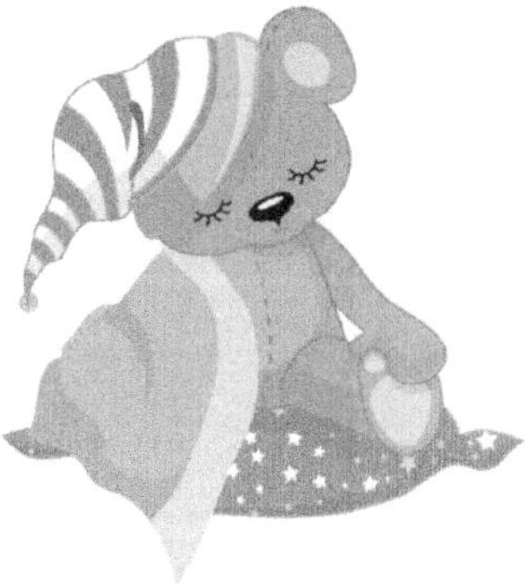

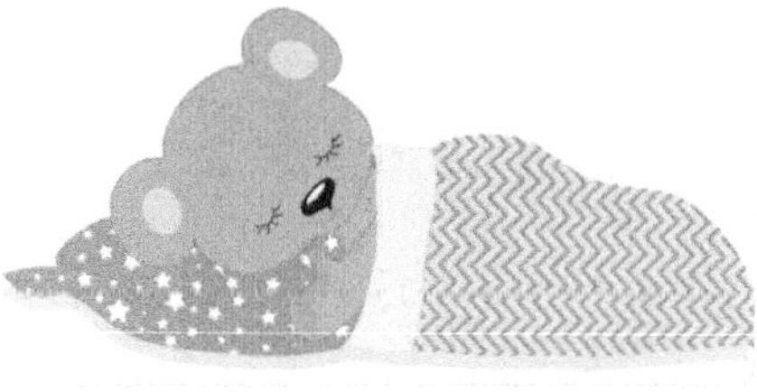

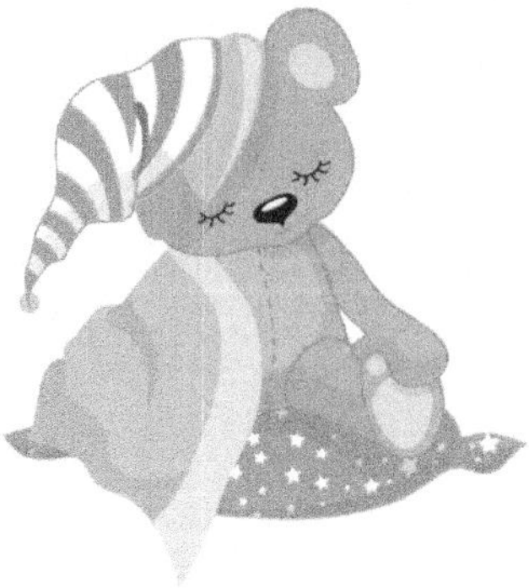

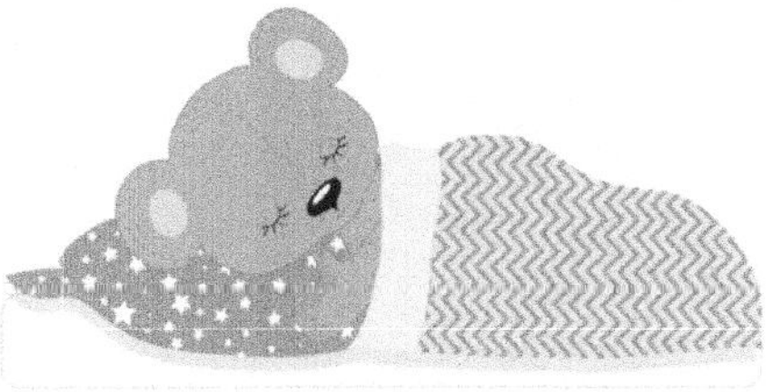

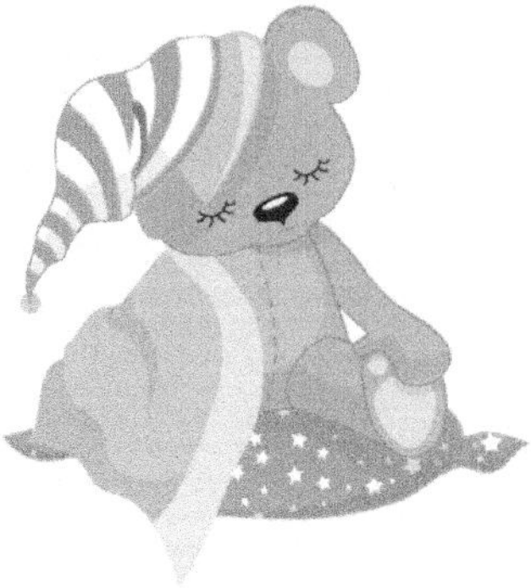

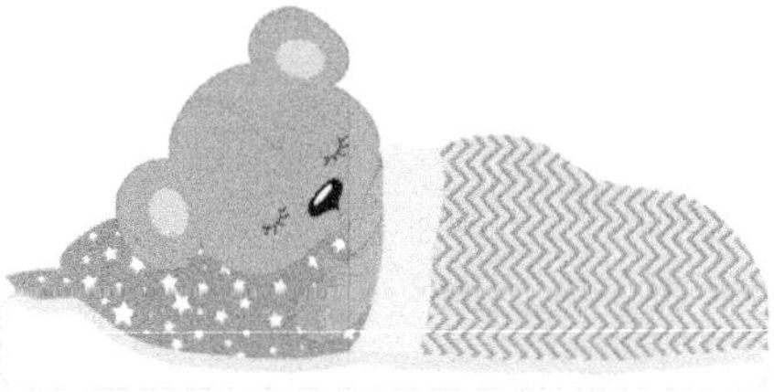

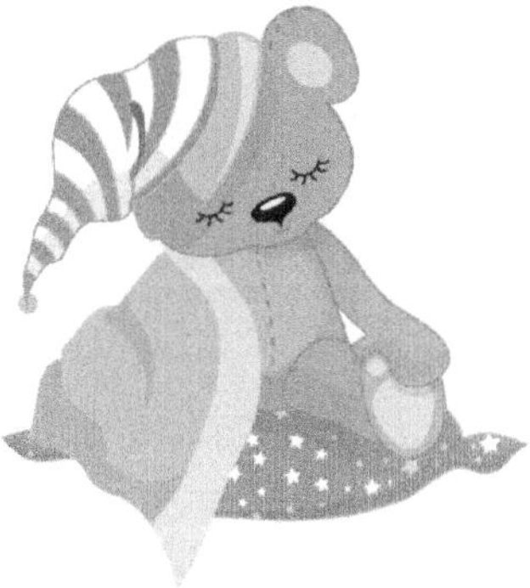

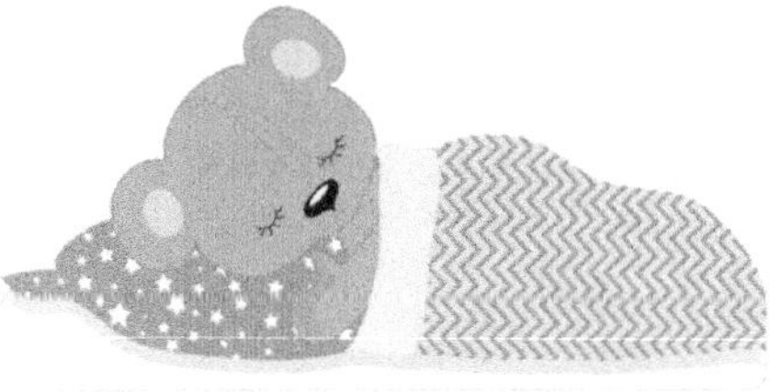

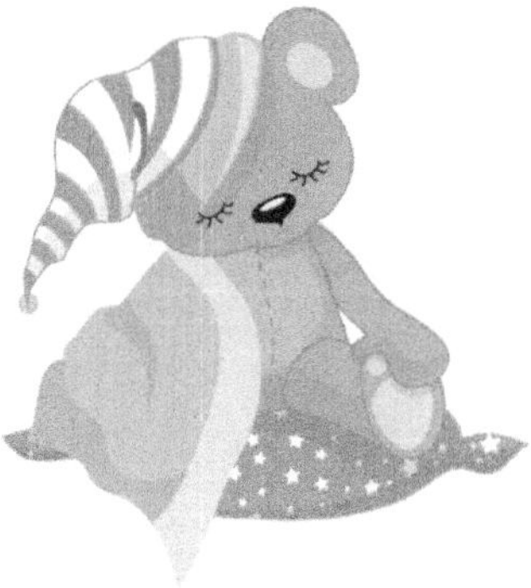

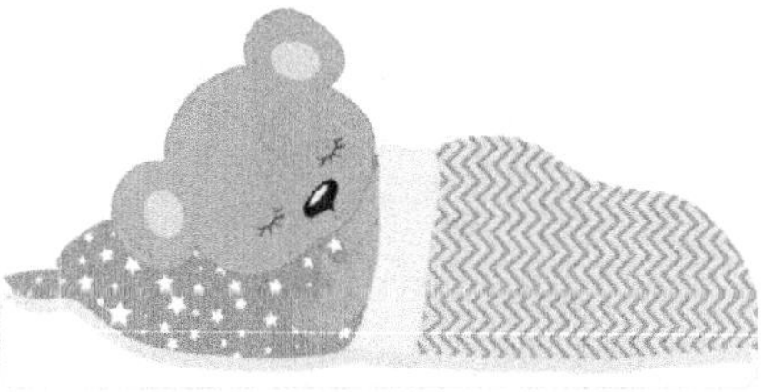

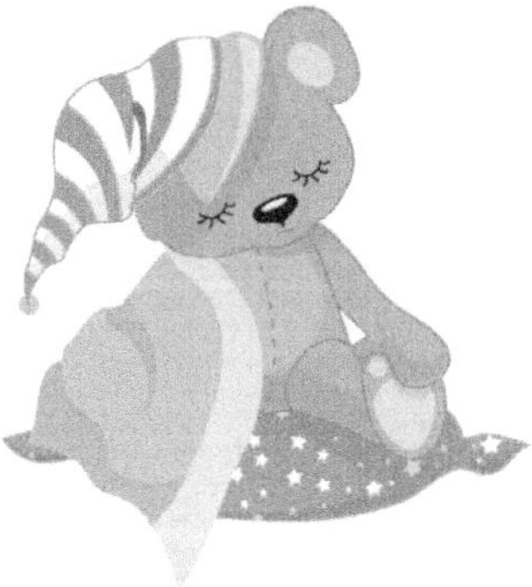

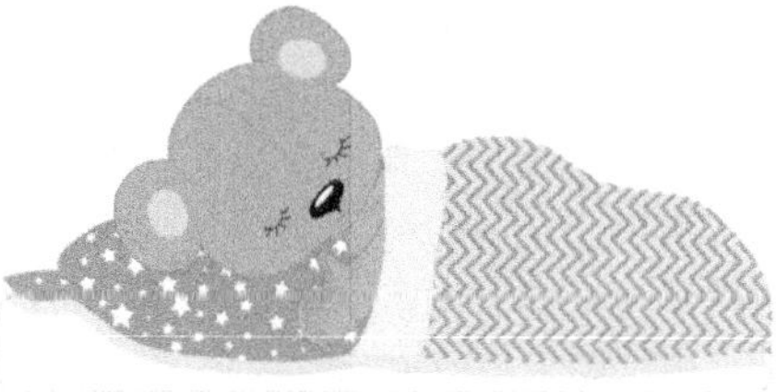

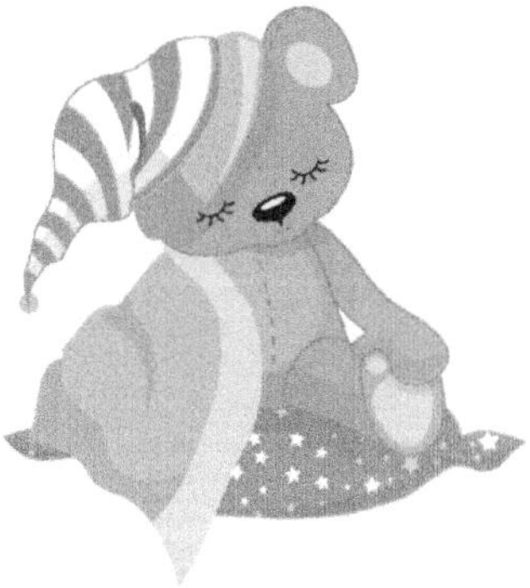

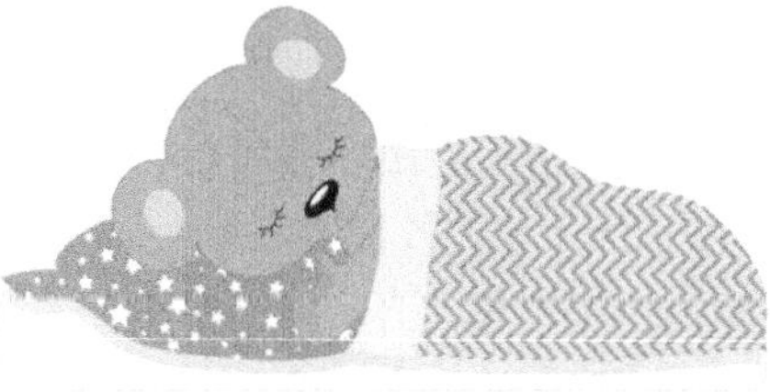

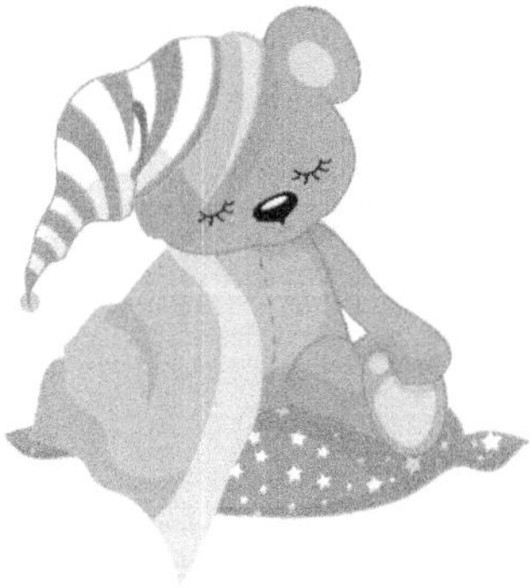

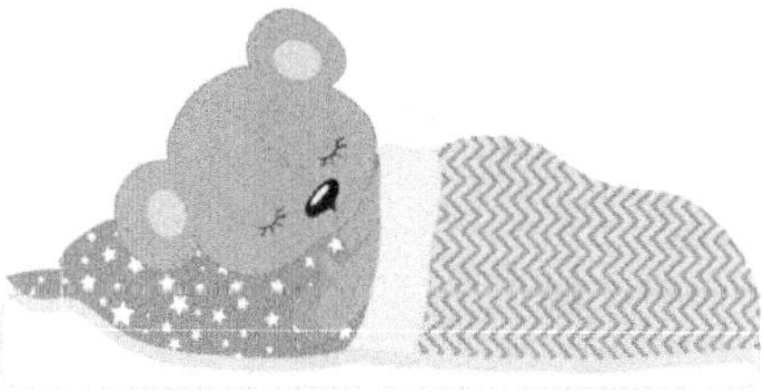

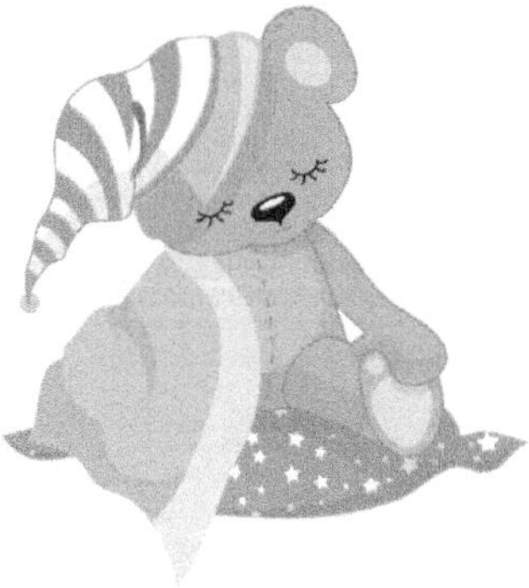

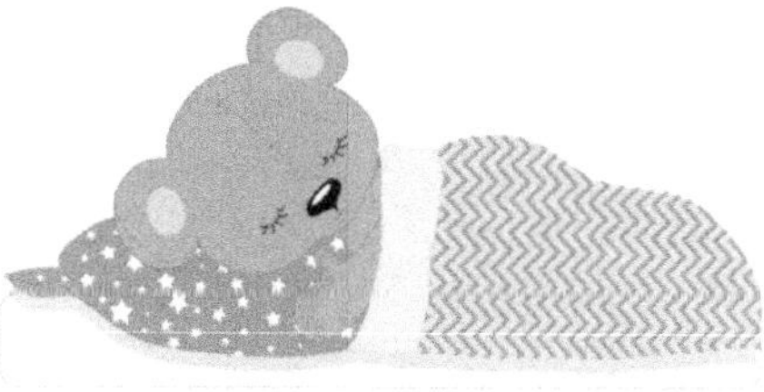

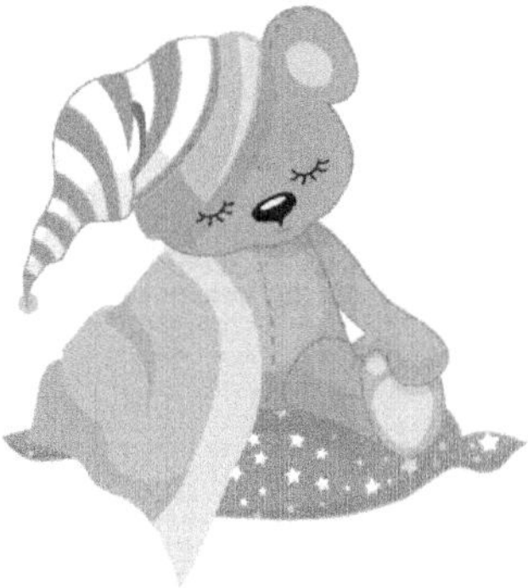

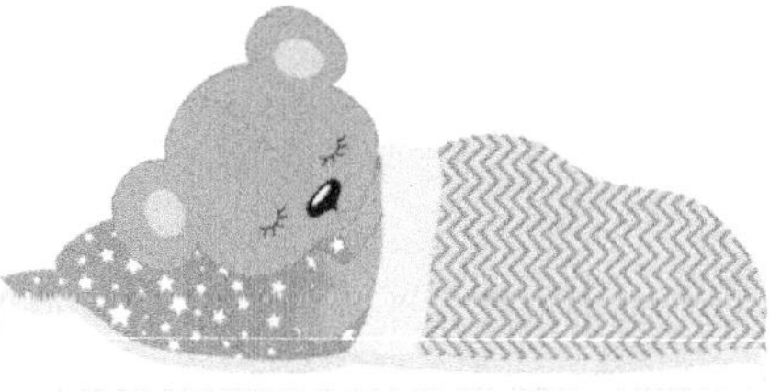

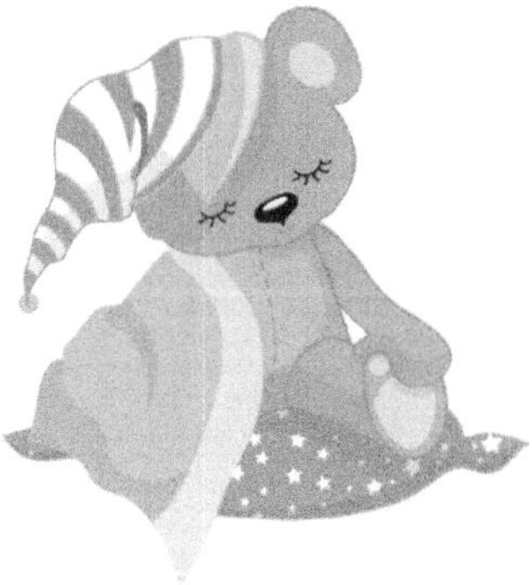

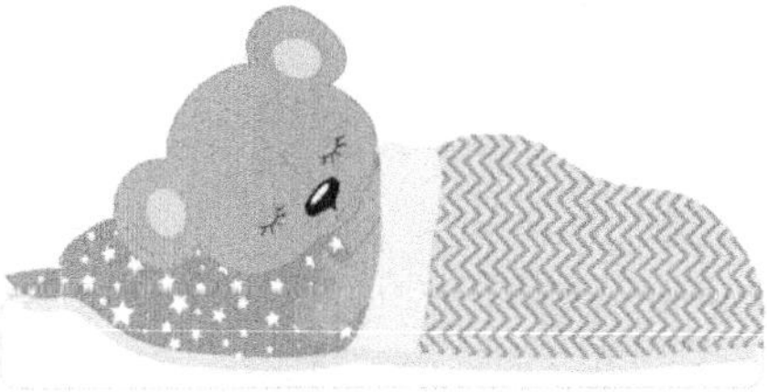

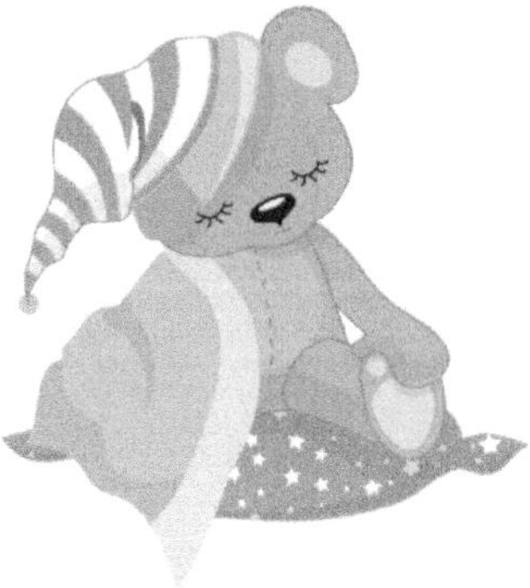

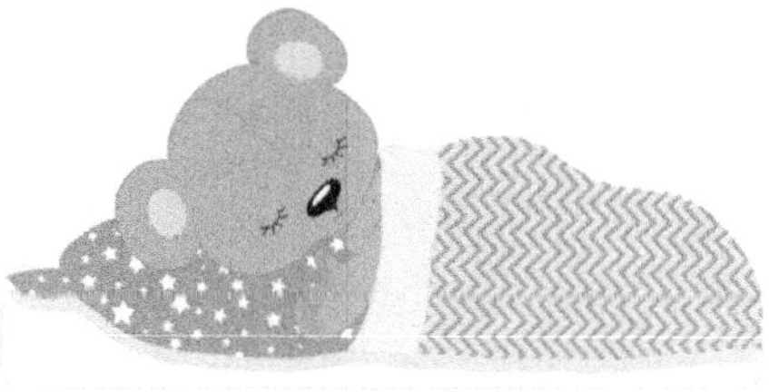

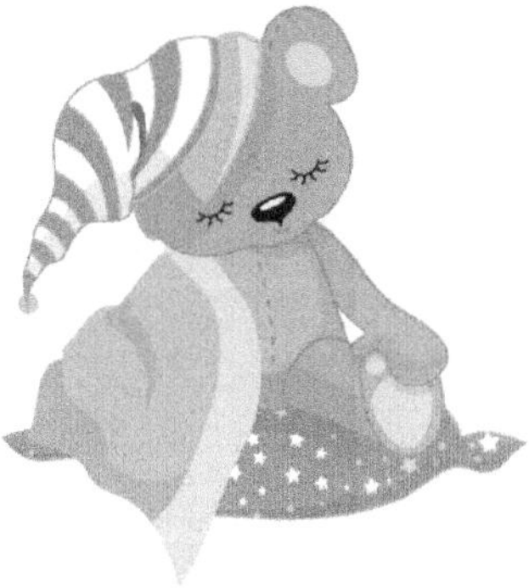

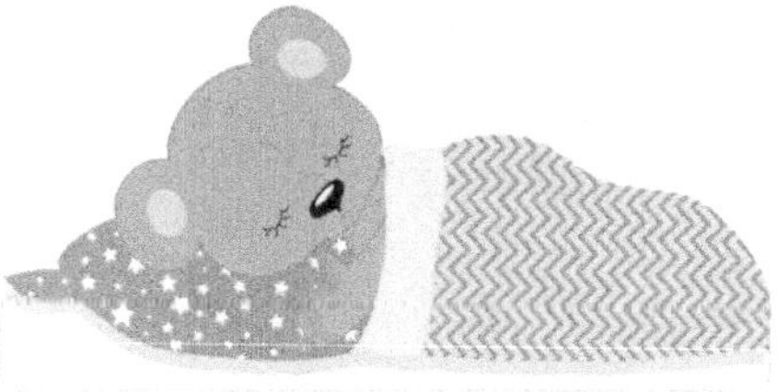

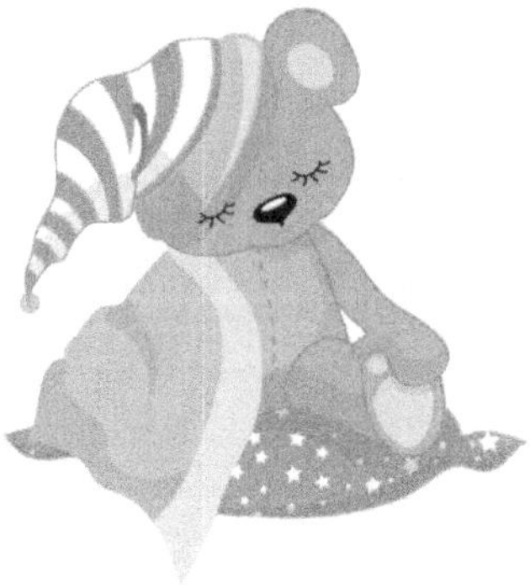

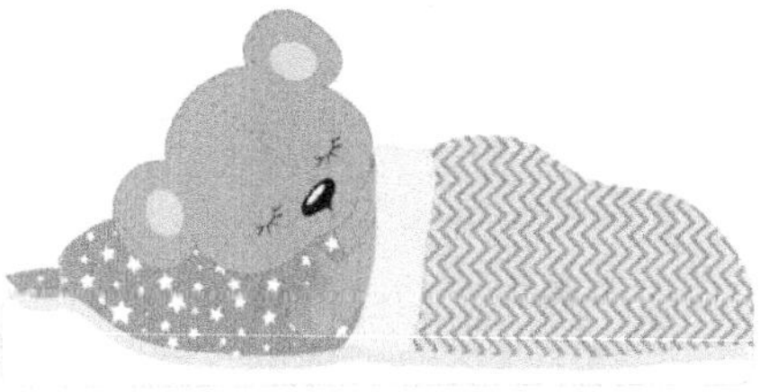

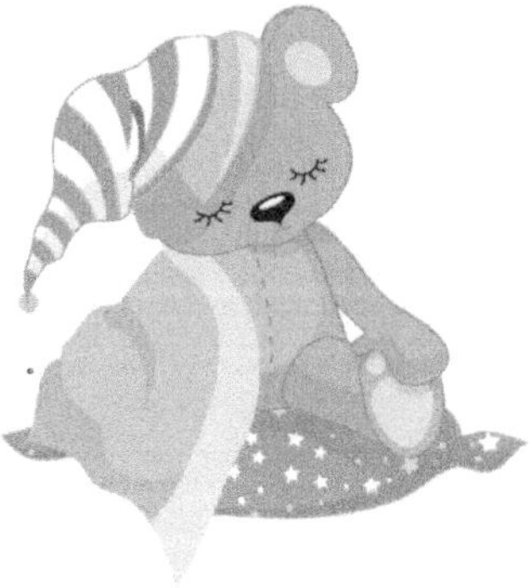

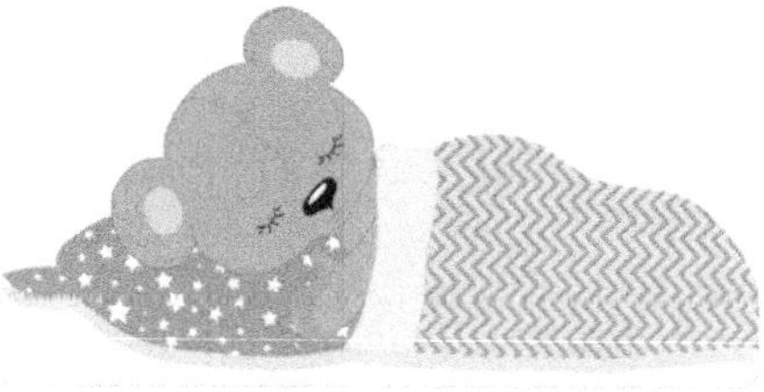

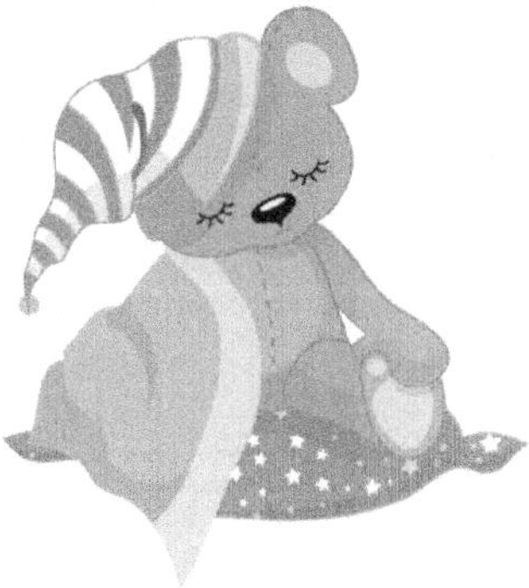

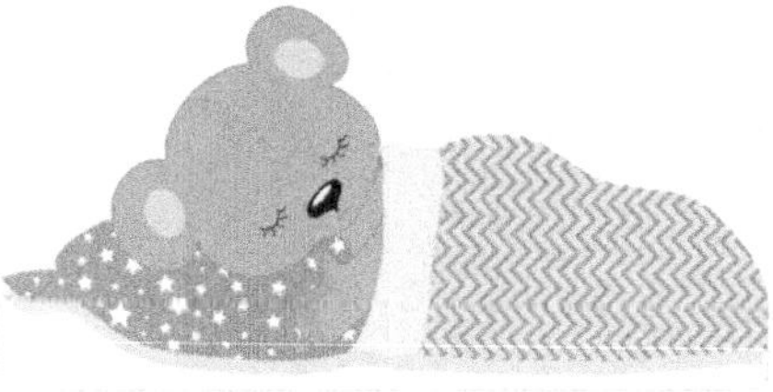

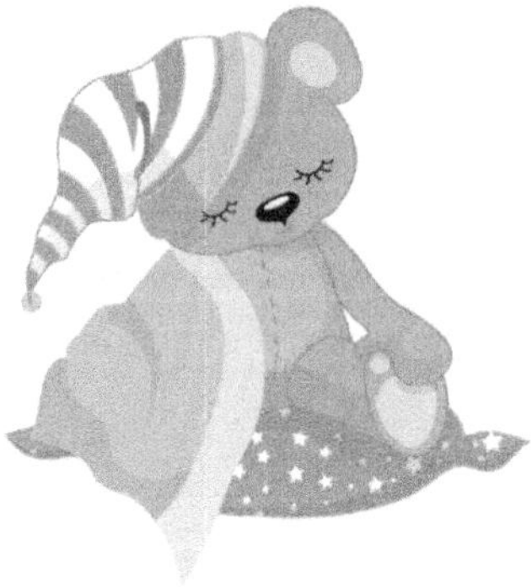

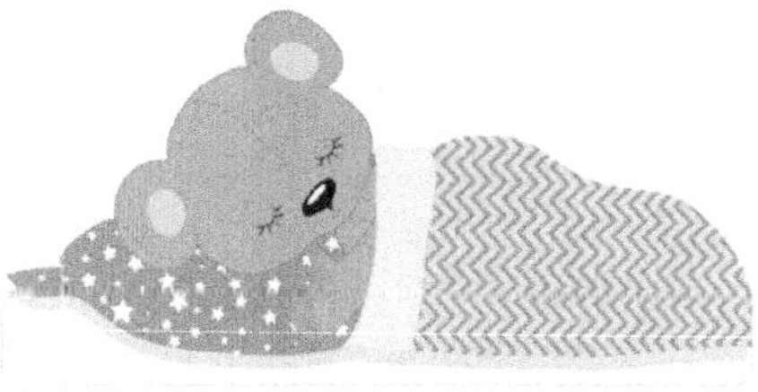

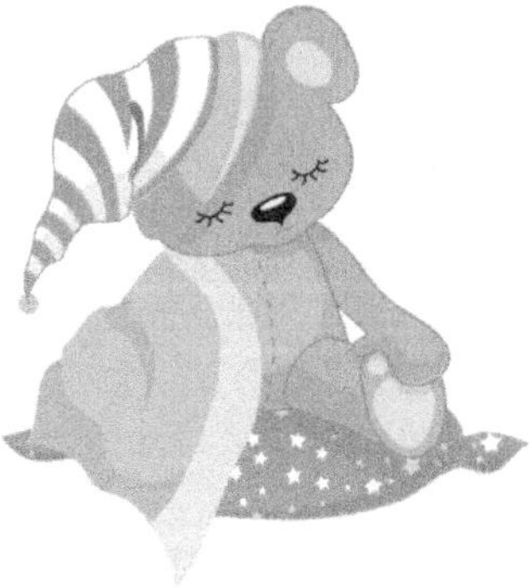

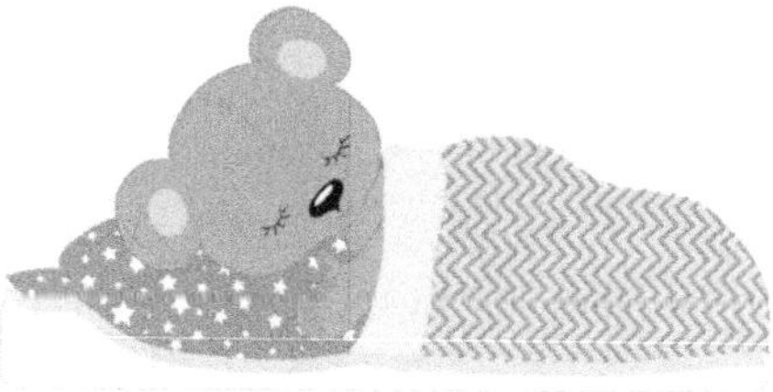

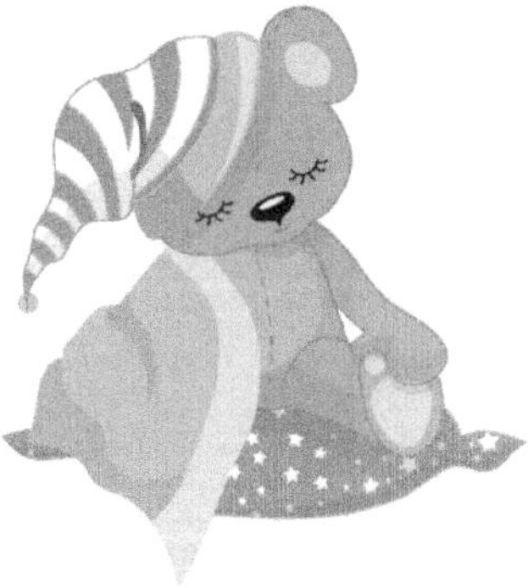

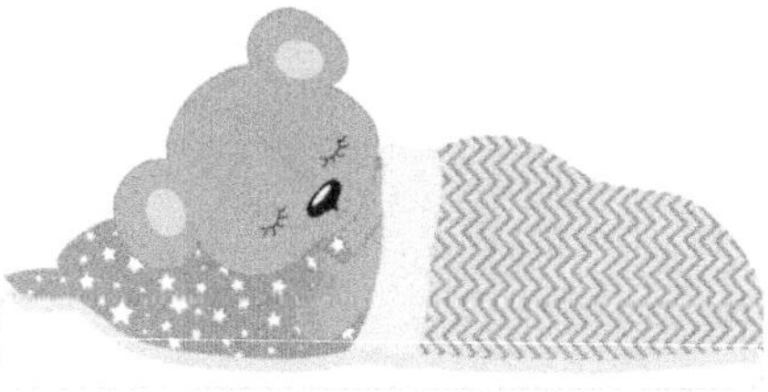

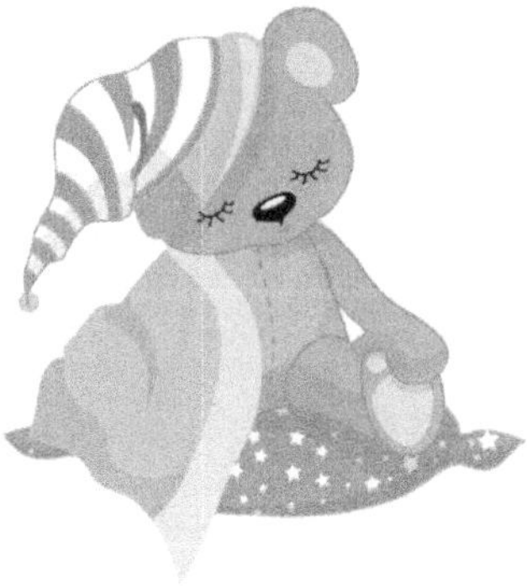

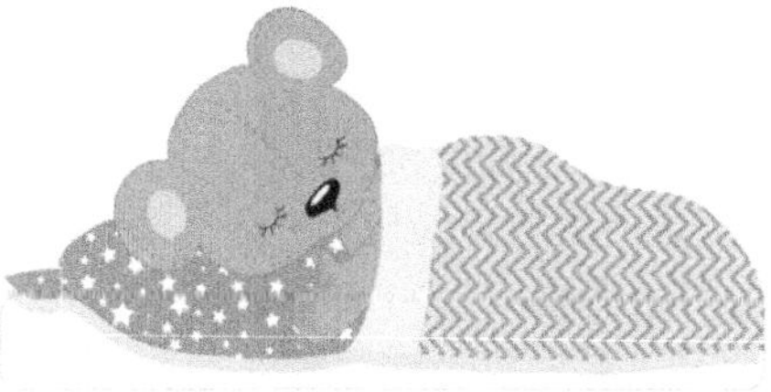

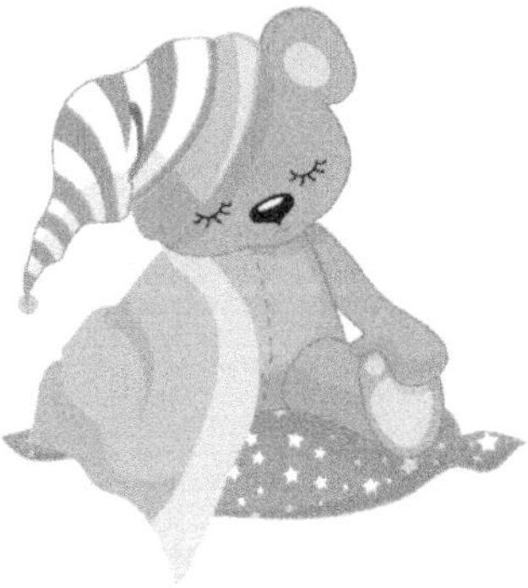

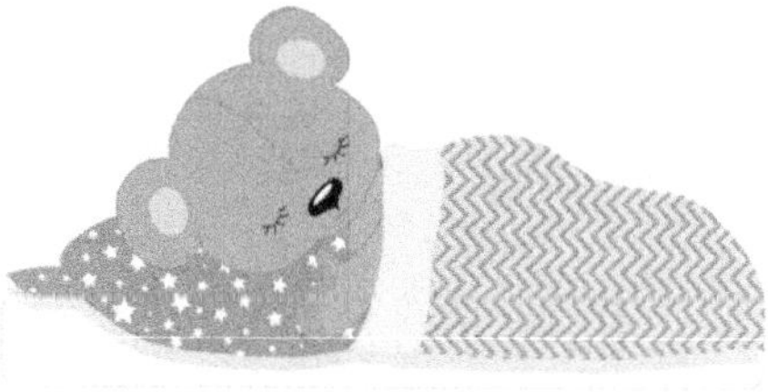

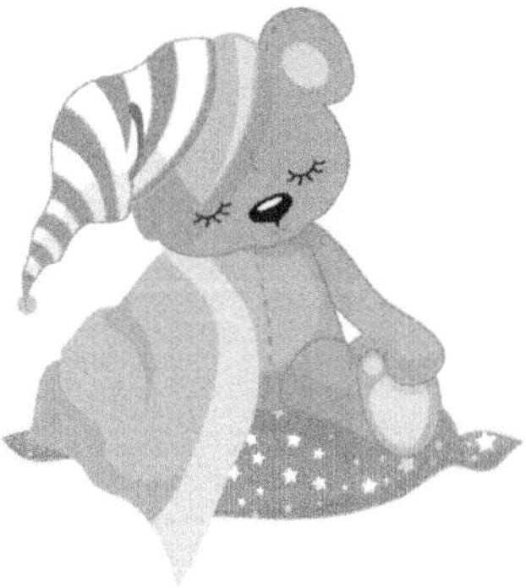

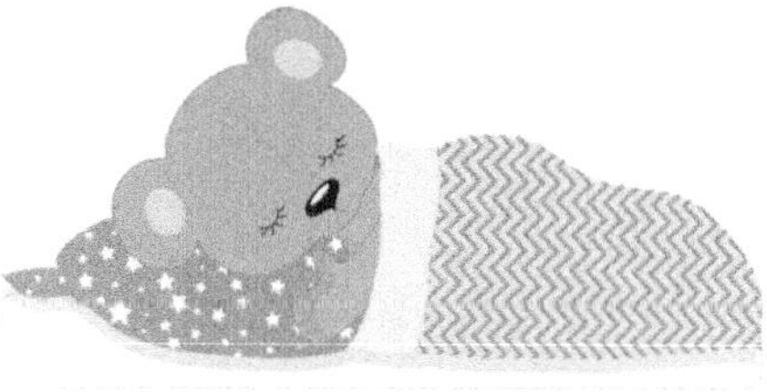

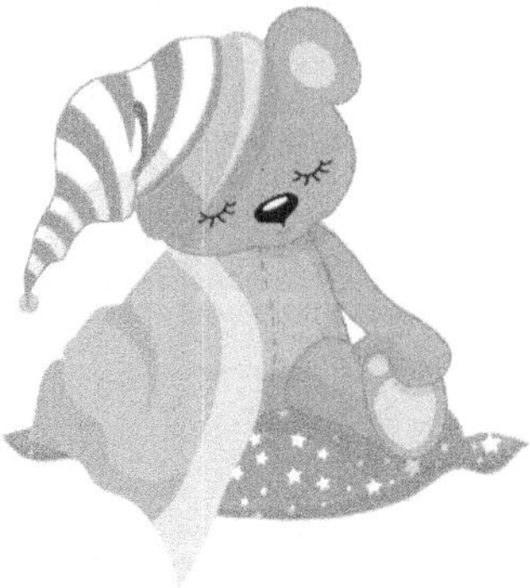

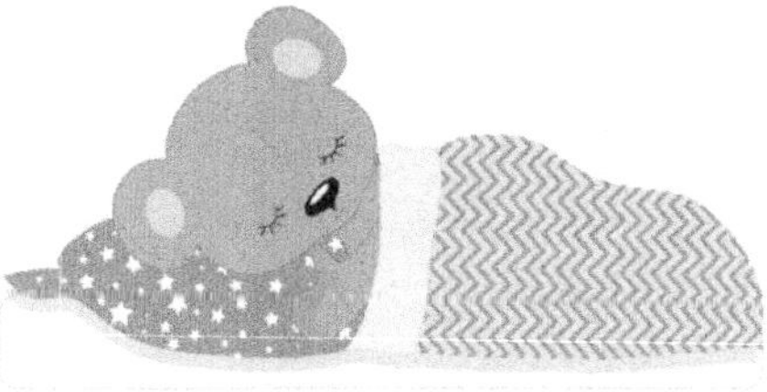

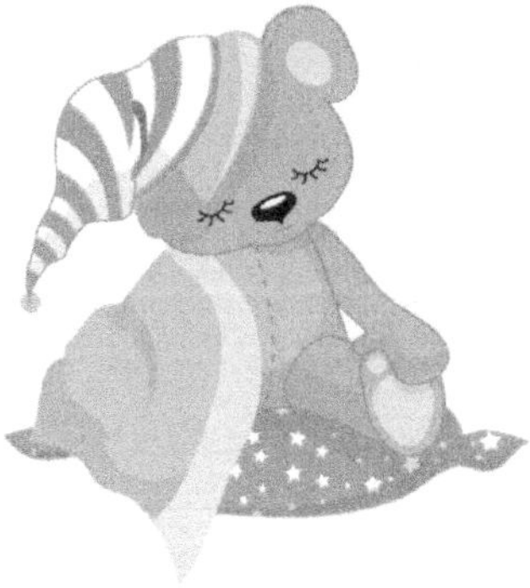

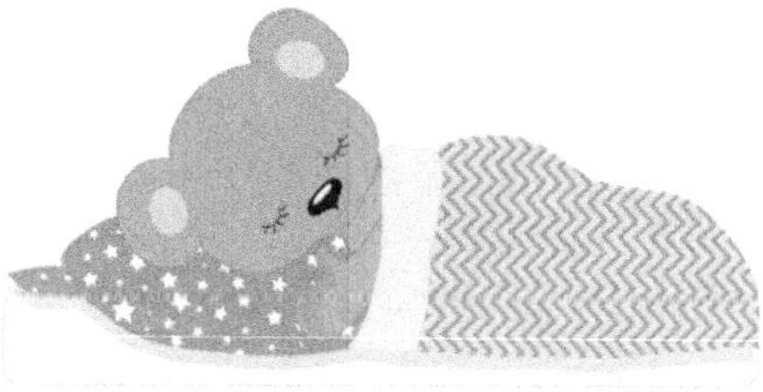

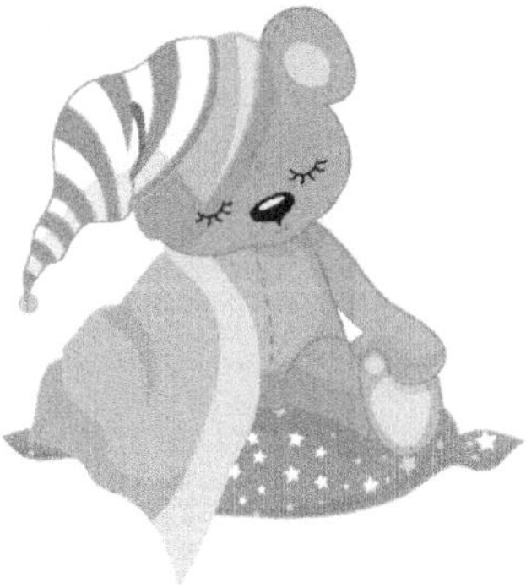

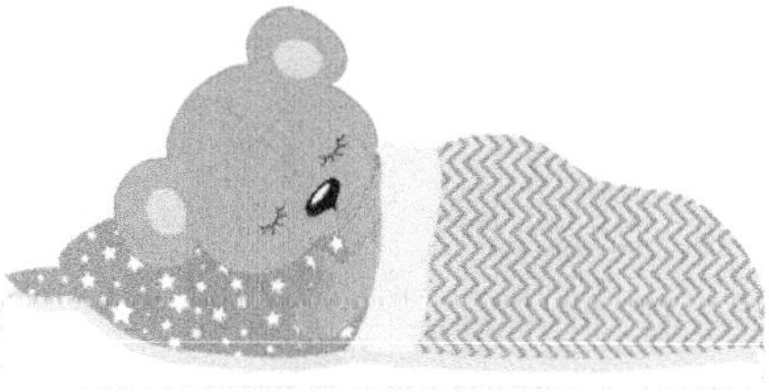

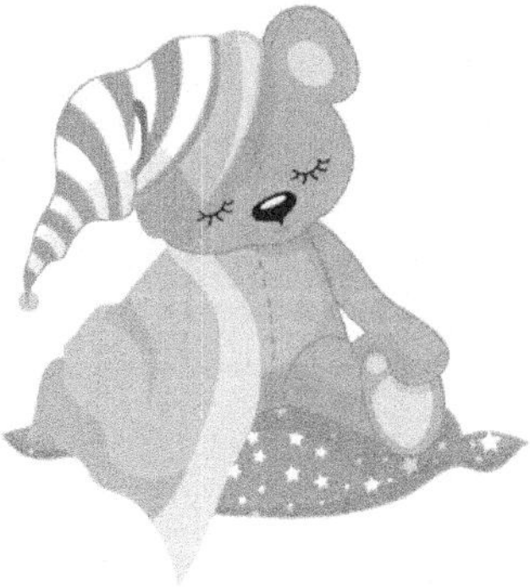

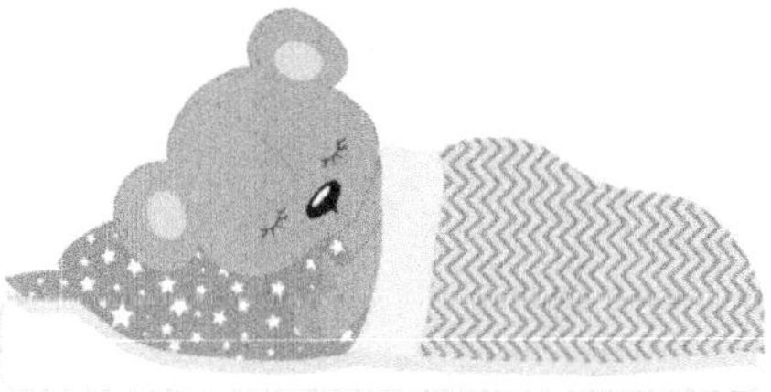

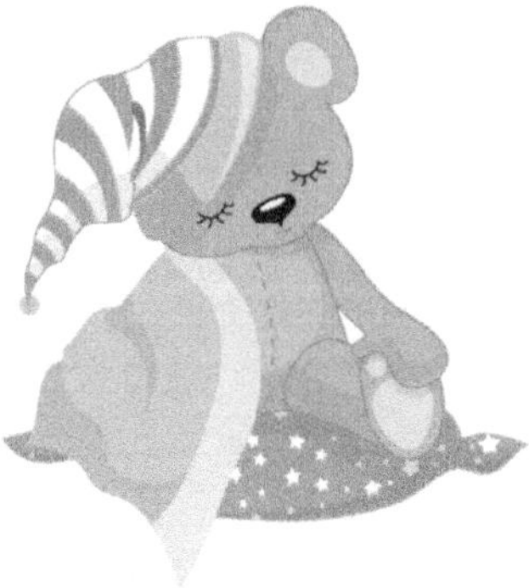

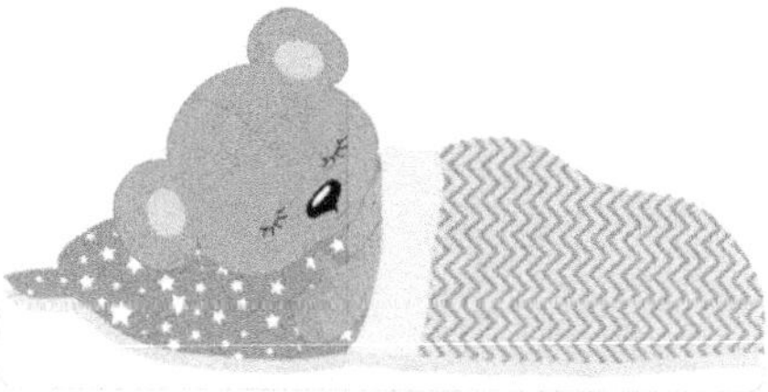

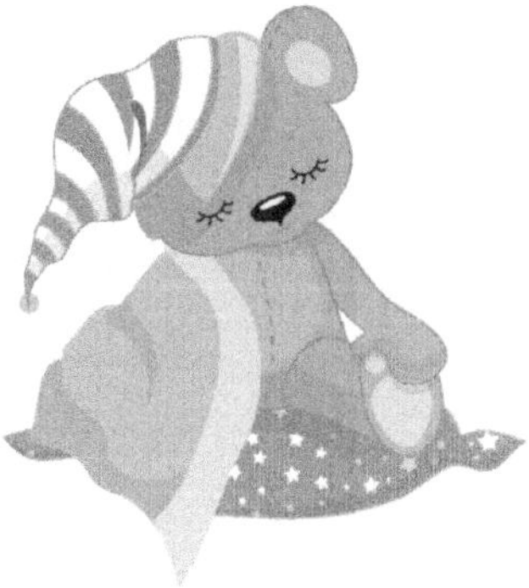

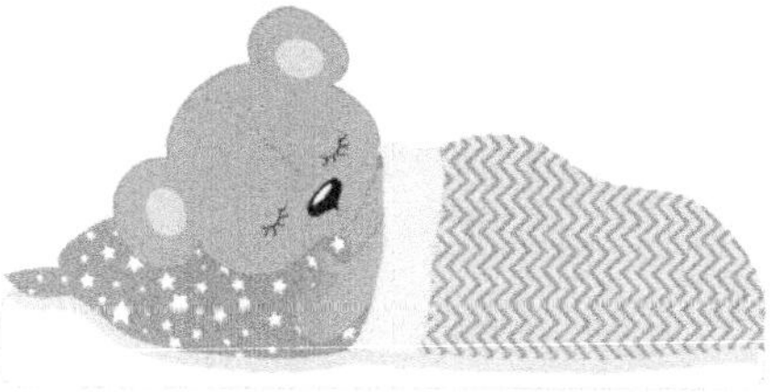

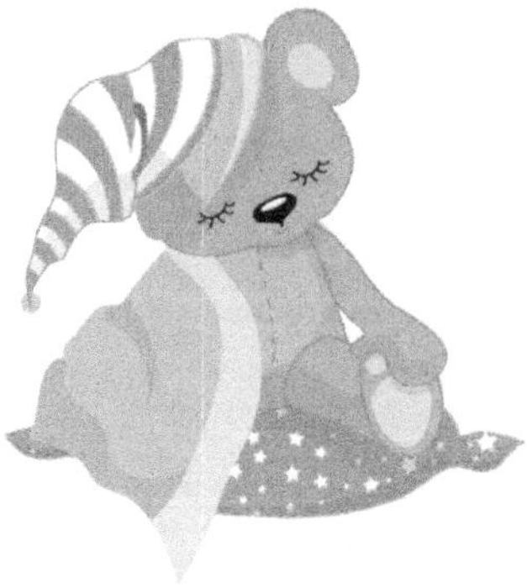

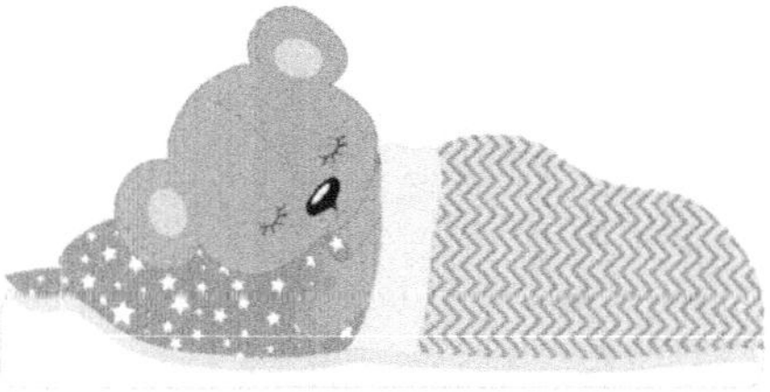

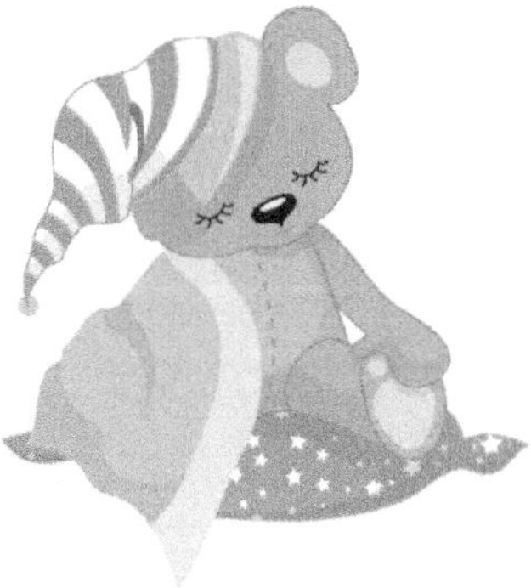

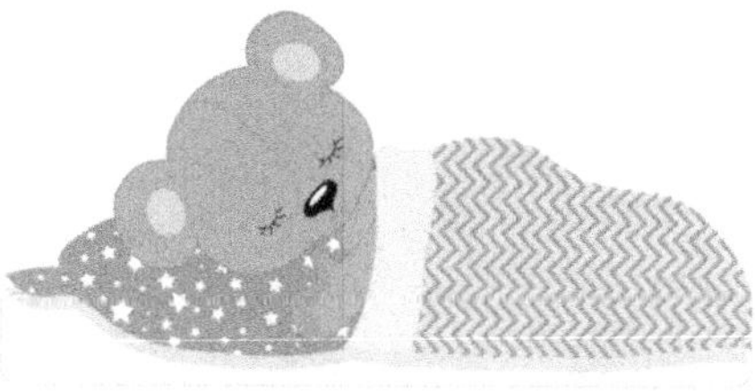

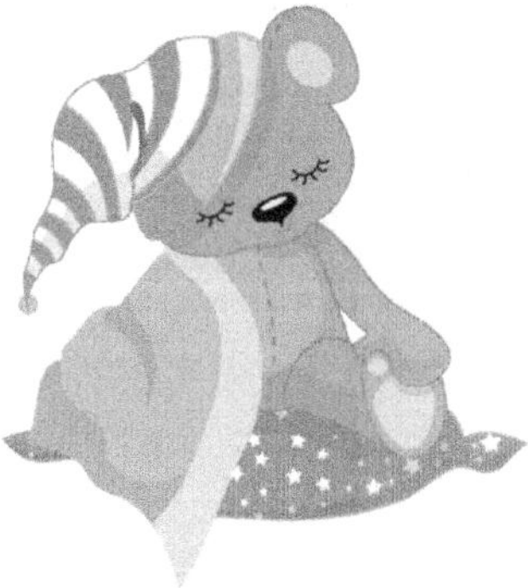

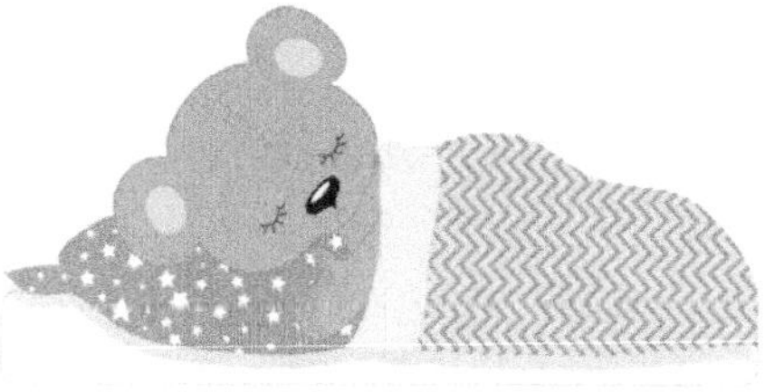

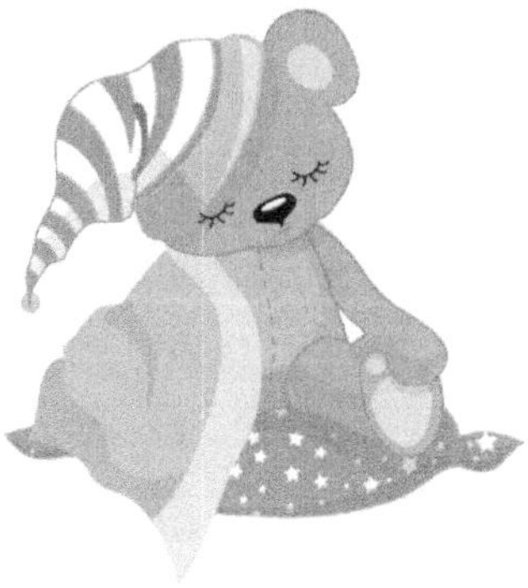

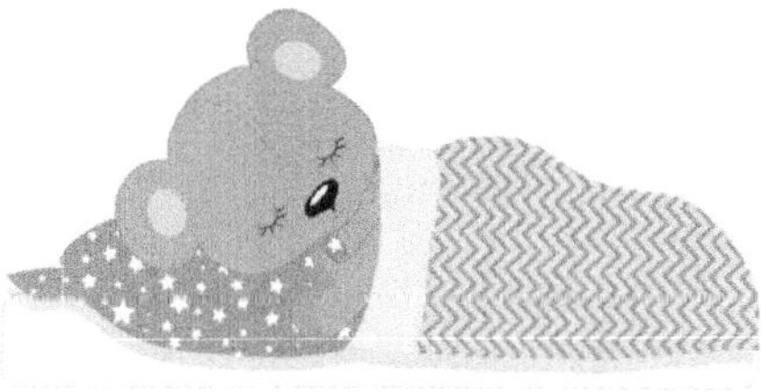

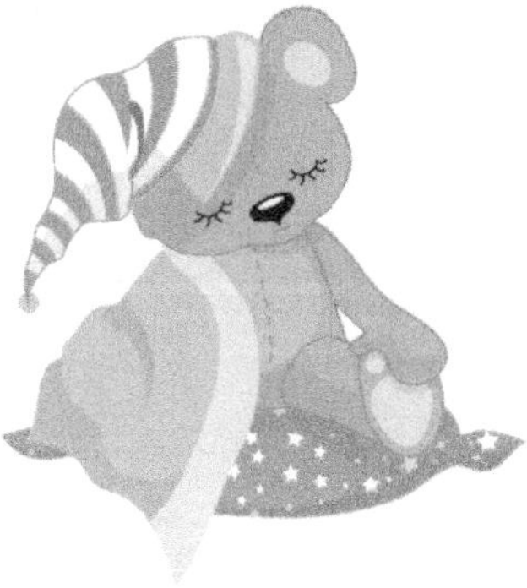

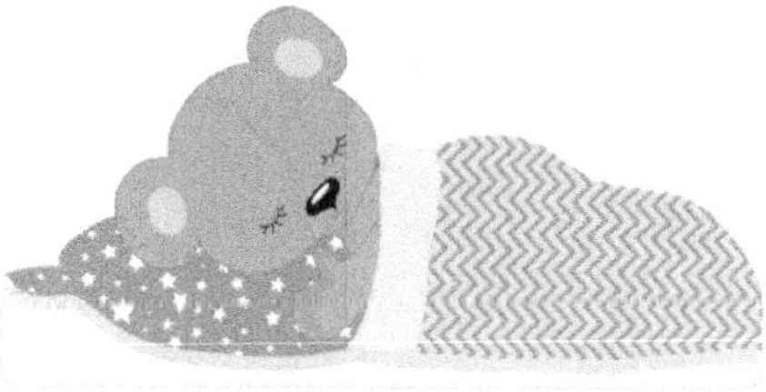

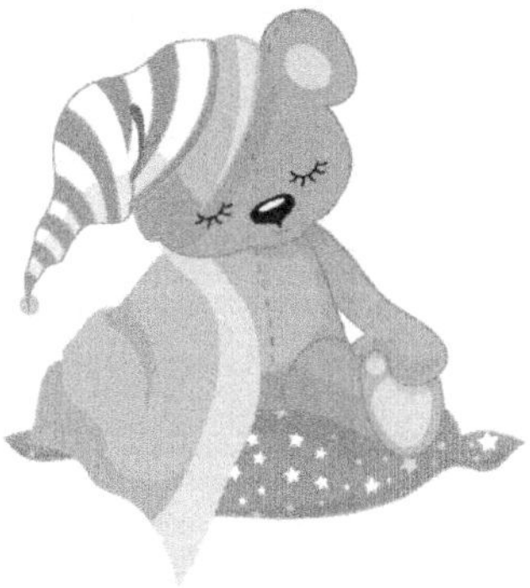

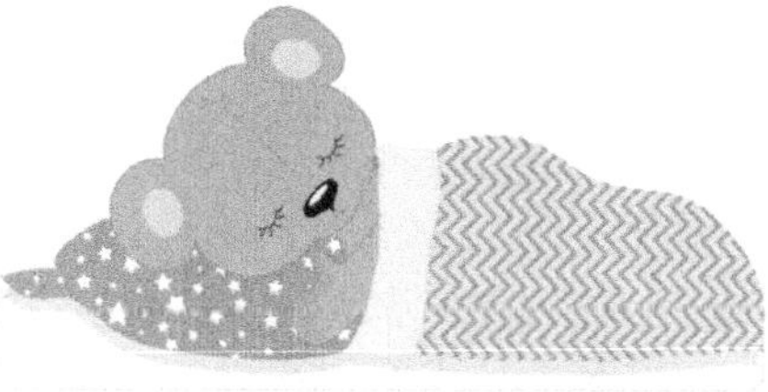

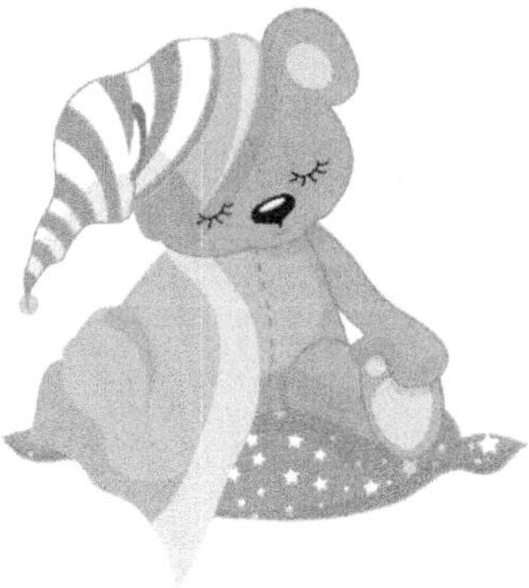

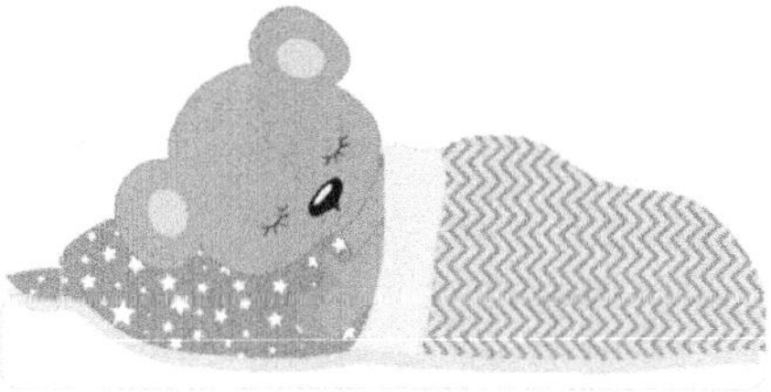

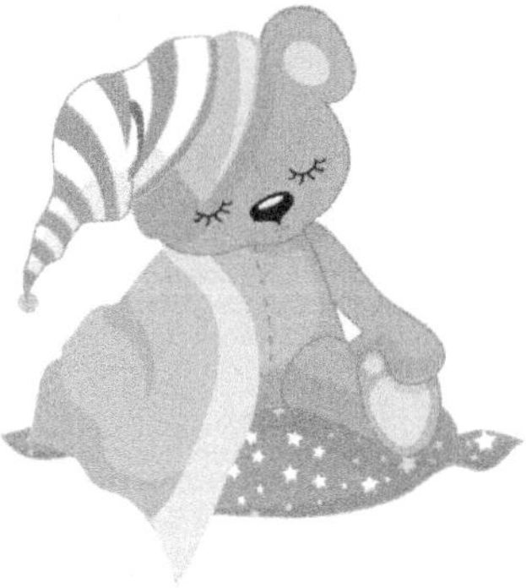

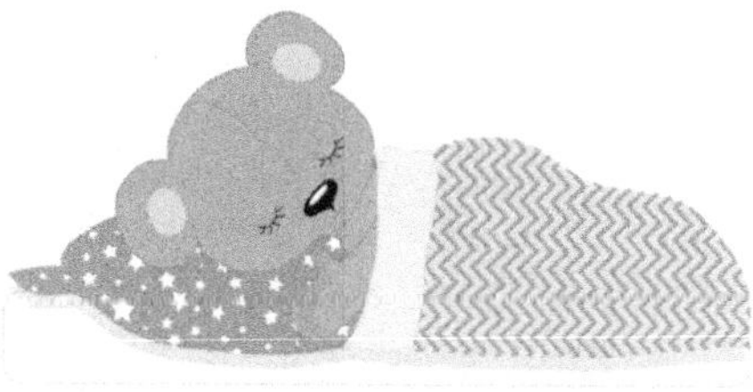

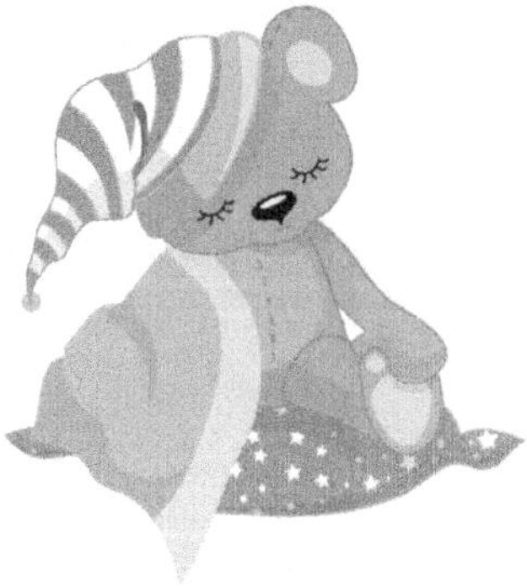

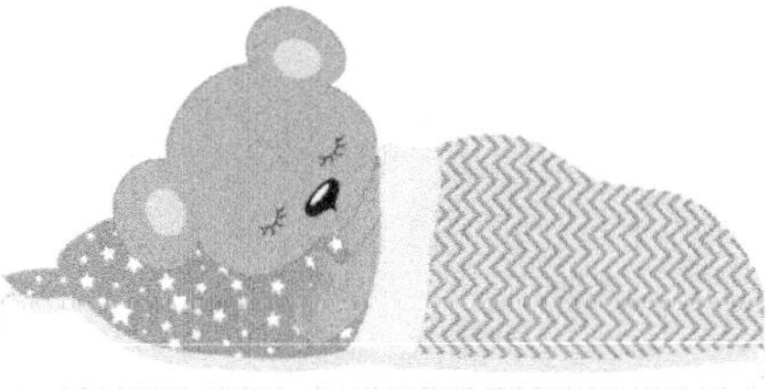

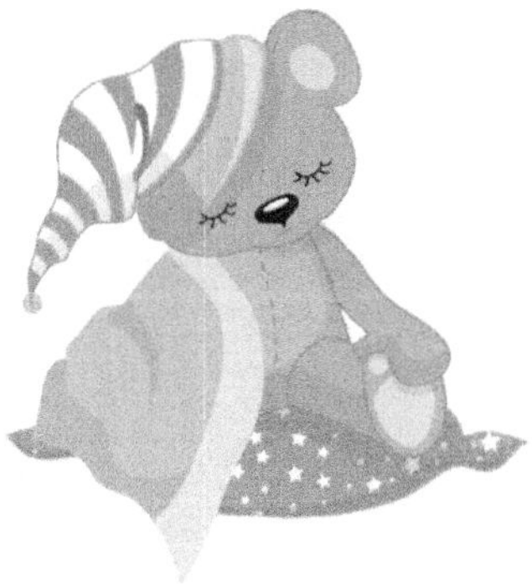

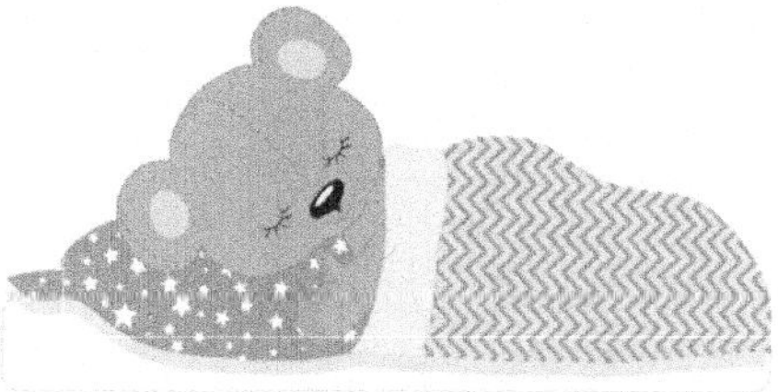

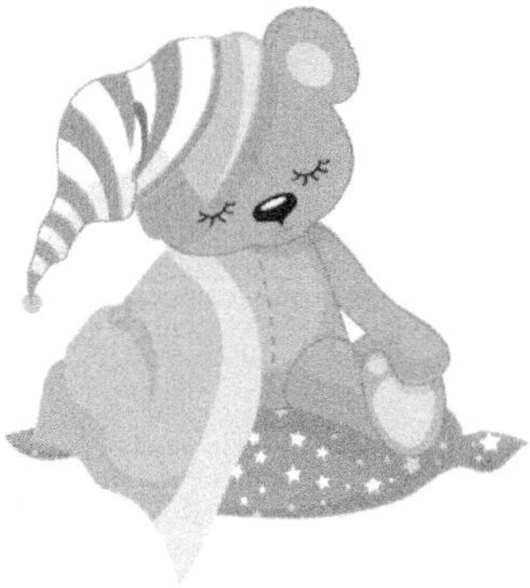

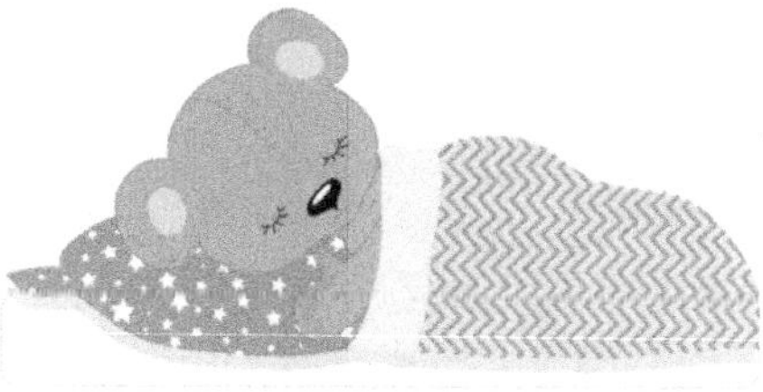

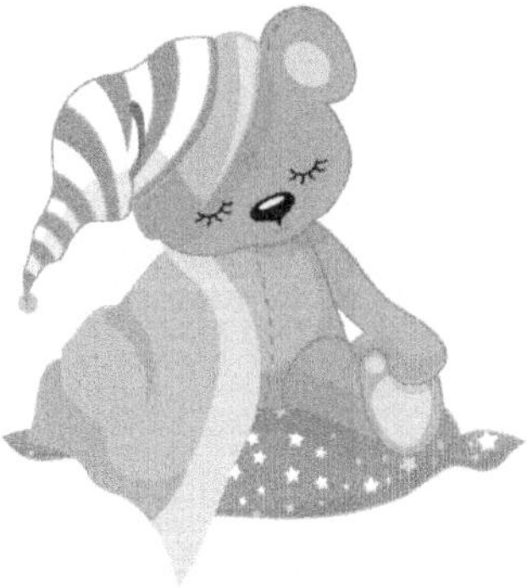

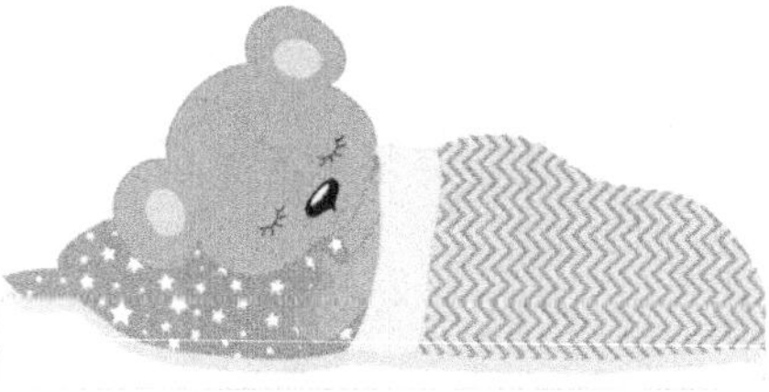

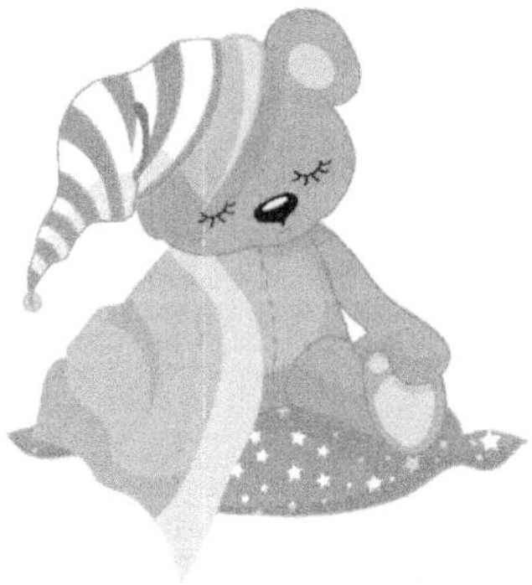

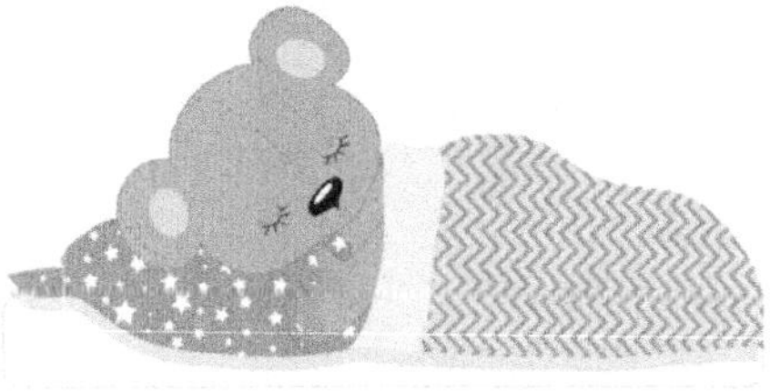

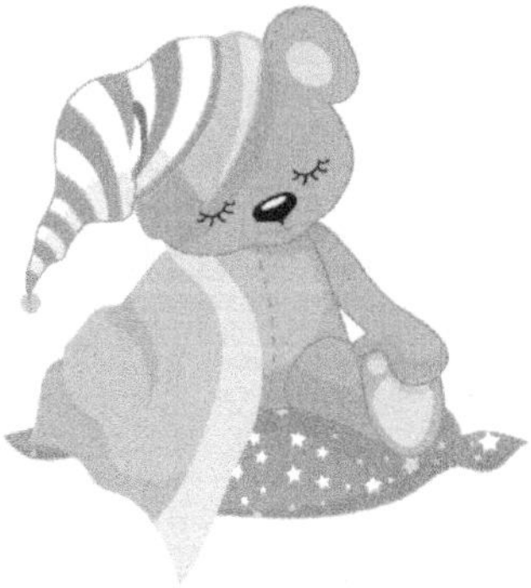

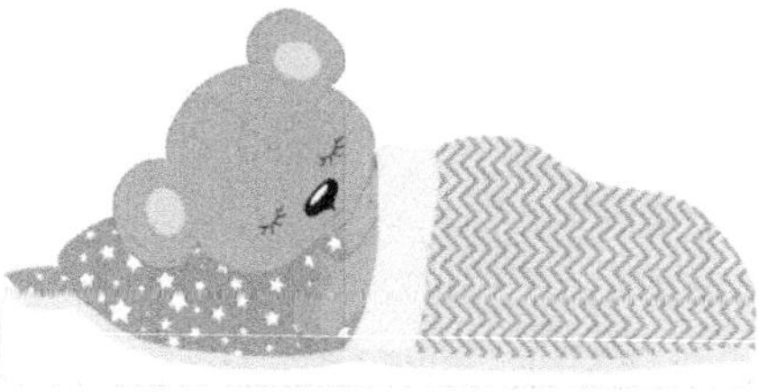

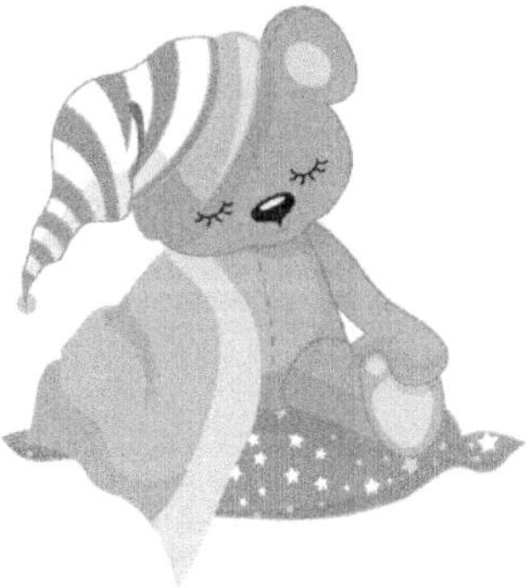

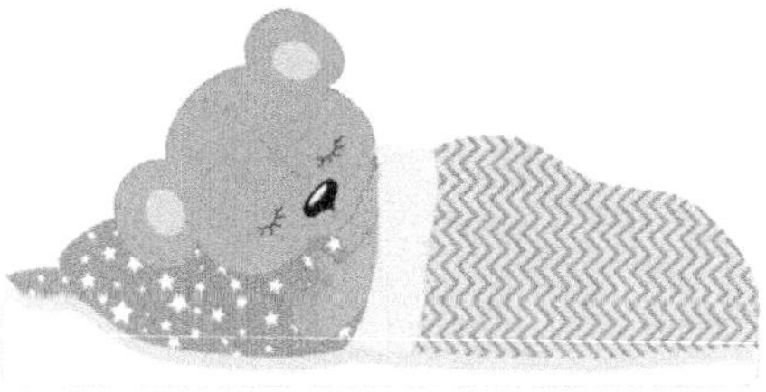

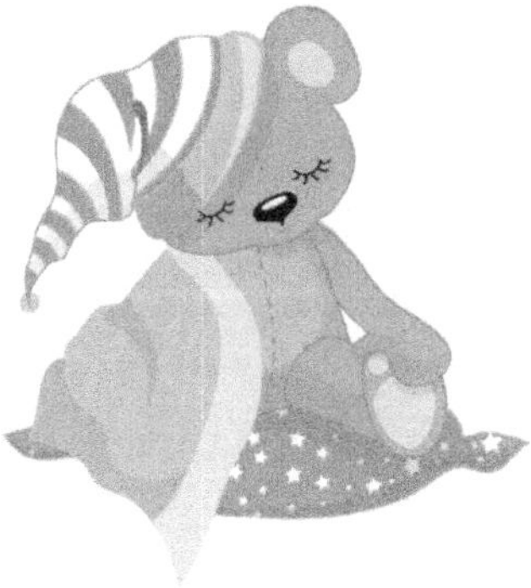

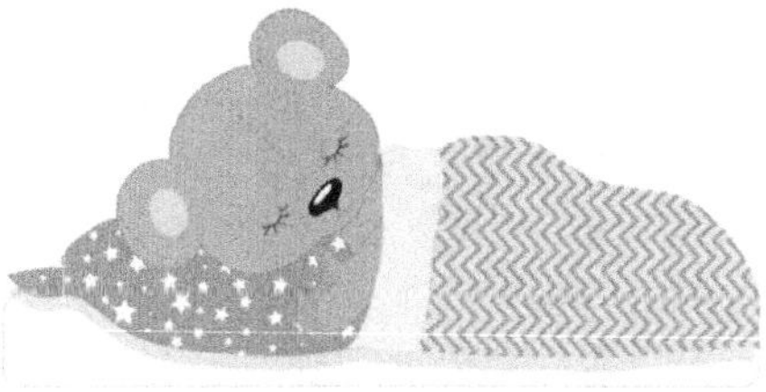

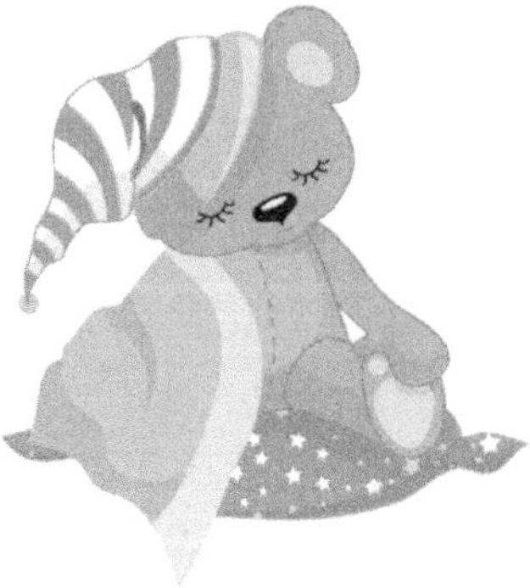

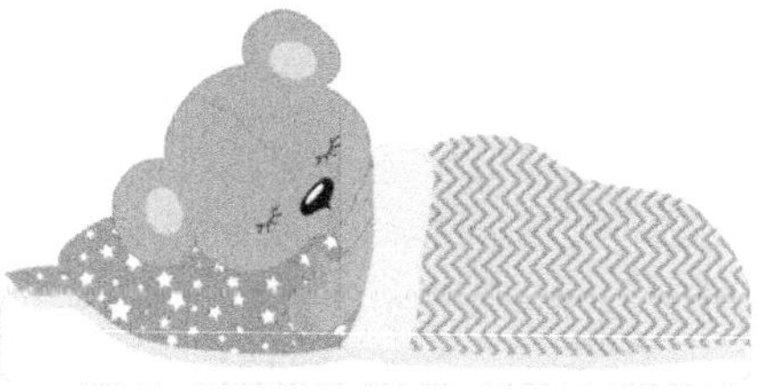

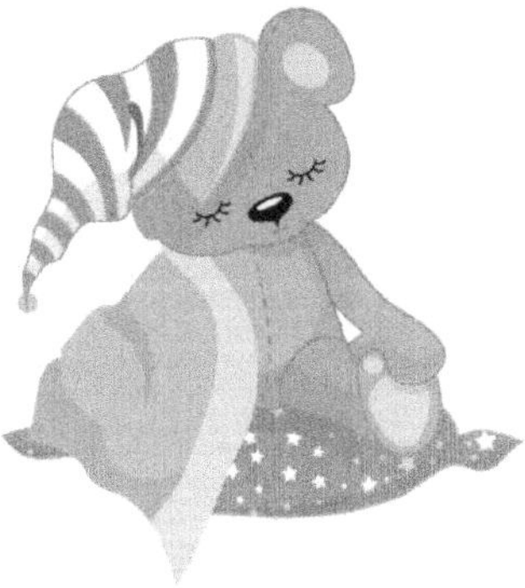

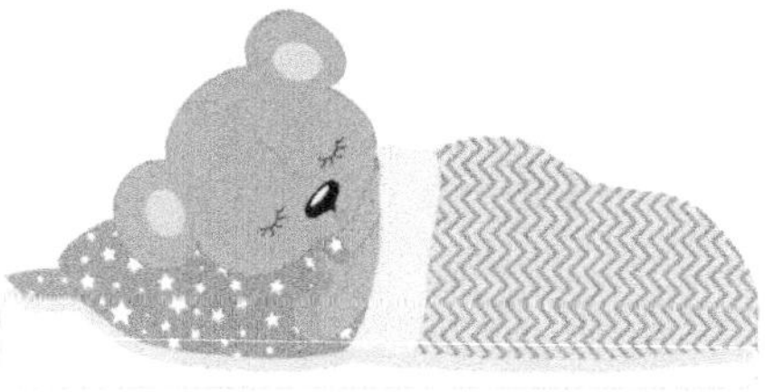

Made in the USA
Monee, IL
19 August 2022

11966384R10069